MEDITERRANEAN AND GLUTEN FREE DIET FOR BEGINNERS

TWO SIMPLE GUIDES AND COOKBOOKS, ONE SPECIFICALLY FOR THOSE WHO WANT TO FOLLOW THE MEDITERRANEAN DIET AND ONE FOR THOSE WHO WANT TO FOLLOW THE GLUTEN-FREE DIET, TO LOSE WEIGHT AND LIVE BETTER (300 RECIPES)

TWO BOOKS IN ONE

By
Riccardo MANZO & Luigi BIANCHI

TABLE OF CONTENS

INTODUCTION

The way we think of the word "diet" today suggests something restrictive and aimed at weight loss. The Mediterranean diet is not far from this but much easier to make. However, it is a heart-healthy eating pattern that contains staple foods used by people living in countries around the Mediterranean Sea such as Greece, Croatia, and Italy. You will find that a plant-based dietary approach rich in vegetables and healthy fats, including olive oil and omega-3 fatty acids from fish, is most emphasized in the meals of citizens of these countries. The Mediterranean diet is known for the benefits it gives to the heart. This diet contains plenty of fruits and vegetables, as well as whole grains, seafood, nuts and legumes, and olive oil. In this diet plan you will be limited in ingesting or avoiding red meat, sugary foods, and dairy products (even if small amounts such as yogurt and cheese are included). Eating this way will allow you to avoid elaborate dishes. The dishes of the Mediterranean diet are very colorful. Traditional proteins such as those derived from chicken can be more of a side dish of the products, which become the main element. One thing you will find that the Mediterranean diet is loved by people is that you can drink red wine in low to moderate quantities. "Moderate" means 5 ounces (oz) or less each day (ie about a glass). However, it should be noted that a glass of wine a day is not mandatory in this meal plan, and if you are not already used to drinking it, it is not the diet that should get you started

BIRTH OF THE MEDITERRANEAN DIET

In the 1950s, Ancel Keys, an American nutritionist, discovered that some diseases were contracted more rarely in the Mediterranean than in the United States. From this observation the hypothesis arose that the Mediterranean diet is able to increase the longevity of those who intend to follow it. In this book, the results of the well-known "Seven Countries Study" were narrated, which for twenty years monitored the nutritional and health conditions of 12,000 people aged between 40 and 60, residing in different countries such as the USA, Japan , former Yugoslavia, Holland and Italy. What was initially observed by Keys' studies confirmed: the Mediterranean diet has been proposed to the whole world as the ideal diet to reduce the incidence of so-called "diseases of well-being" Since the early 1970s, this diet and its eating habits have also been introduced in the United States. Cereals, vegetables, fruits, fish and olive oil have been presented as an alternative to a diet too high in fat, protein and sugar. To summarize all the principles of the Mediterranean diet, in the 1990s the design of a "pyramid" was created which shows the distribution, frequency and quantity of foods throughout the day. In particular, at its base there are the foods to be consumed several times a day, while at the apex the foods to be limited are indicated..

BENEFITS OF THE MEDITERRANEAN DIET

The Mediterranean diet is particularly known for the benefits it brings to heart health and for the fact that it reduces the risk of heart disease, in part by lowering LDL ("bad") cholesterol levels and reducing mortality from cardiovascular disease. . The Mediterranean diet has also been credited with reducing the likelihood of certain cancers, such as breast cancer, as well as conditions such as Parkinson's and Alzheimer's. Some empirical data also shows that this diet improves life and protects people with type 2 diabetes. Following the Mediterranean diet program improves glycemic control in those people who have already been diagnosed with type 2 diabetes, resulting in better management. . . of the disease. Also, considering that people with diabetes are more likely to have cardiovascular disease, following this diet improves their heart health. This has also been confirmed by established scientific journals. Finally, those who follow this diet eat about nine servings of fruit and vegetables a day. The disease-fighting antioxidants that are released with these foods reduce the risk so that people following the diet have a lower risk of getting sick. So, as established scientists and dieticians point out, there is no certainty as to whether antioxidants or other compounds (or healthy eating patterns in general) are responsible for these benefits.

HOW TO MANAGE THIS DIET

The Mediterranean diet is mainly focused on the correct choice of food, while the caloric aspect plays a secondary role. Portion control and moderation are always an essential element for the correct application of this diet. Indicatively, an adult man would need about 2,500 calories per day, of which 55-65% should come from carbohydrates, 20-30% from lipids and only 10-15% from proteins. The most important principles of the Mediterranean diet are contained in the following guidelines:

1. Greater consumption of vegetable proteins than animal ones
2. Reduction of saturated (animal) fats compared to unsaturated vegetable fats (olive oil)
3. Reduction of the general quantity
4. Increase of complex carbohydrates and strong reduction of simple ones

5. High intake of dietary fiber, great moderation of cholesterol intake
The consumption of white meat higher than the red one, however, is to be limited to once or twice a week. This is also because the diet involves a greater consumption of fish and legumes. Desserts are only allowed on special occasions
The Mediterranean diet also includes a drastic reduction in the consumption of: sausages, super alcohol, white sugar, butter, fatty cheeses, mayonnaise, white salt, margarine, beef and pork (especially fatty cuts), lard and coffee.

PIRAMIDE DELLA DIETA MEDITERRANEA

L'immagine mostra la Piramide Alimentare della Dieta Mediterranea rivisitata secondo canoni più moderni. Indica semplicemente quali cibi mangiare giornalmente, settimanalmente, mensilmente e sporadicamente e le loro quantità raccomandate.

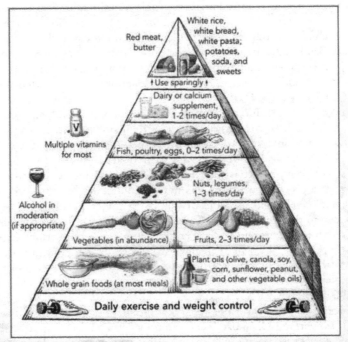

AUTHOR'S NOTE: Calorie indications are for one serve
This book has given you all the information you need to do this diet correctly and do it right. It is essential to understand what you are getting into when you embark on this diet, and this book gave you valuable information that you can use to your advantage and avoid the problems that can come with this diet. You want to stay healthy and make sure that your body can do what it needs to do. As with anything, we emphasize that if something seems wrong or unnatural, you will need to see a doctor to make sure you are safe and that your body can handle this diet. Use the knowledge in this book to get amazing recipes and learn directions for excellent meals for yourself. Consult your doctor before to starting new diet.

1 GINGER CHICKEN TOASTED SESAME GINGER CHICKEN

Servings: 4   **Cook Time: 15Min**   **Prep Time 10 Min**

INGREDIENTS:

- ✓ 1 Tablespoon
- ✓ Toasted Sesame
- ✓ Ginger Seasoning (or toasted sesame seeds
- ✓ Garlic, onion powder
- ✓ Red pepper
- ✓ Ground ginger

- ✓ Salt
- ✓ Pepper
- ✓ Llemon
- ✓ 1 1/2 lbs. boneless, skinless chicken breast
- ✓ 4 teaspoons Olive Oil

DIRECTIONS:

- ➢ On a clean, dry cutting board put the chicken breasts.
- ➢ Softly flatten the chicken breasts to the approx. thickness of 3/8
- ➢ (Use a beef hammer or a frying pans backside)
- ➢ Dust with some seasoning.
- ➢ Heat the Olive Oil over medium-high flame in a big, nonstick frying pan.
- ➢ Add the chicken and cook on one side for about 7-8 minutes

- ➢ (Uuntil a beautiful crust has created ,it will be mildly orange)
- ➢ Turn the chicken softly and cook on the other side for a further 5-6 minutes
- ➢ (Before the chicken is thoroughly cooked)
- ➢ Serve hot or cooled over salad with your favorite side dish
- ➢ Makes about 4 servings.

NUTRITION INFORMATION: 310 kcal Protein: 16.14 g Fat: 10.64 g Carbohydrates: 36.65 g

2 TASTY AND TENDER FISH TACOS

Servings: 4   **Cook Time: 15Min**   **Prep Time 15 Min**

INGREDIENTS:

- ✓ 2 teaspoons Olive Oil (or oil)
- ✓ Fresh garlic
- ✓ 1 capful (1 Tablespoon)
- ✓ Southwestern Seasoning or Phoenix Sunrise
- ✓ Cumin
- ✓ Garlic
- ✓ Cilantro

- ✓ Red pepper
- ✓ Onion
- ✓ Parsley
- ✓ Paprika
- ✓ Salt & pepper (or low sodium taco seasoning)
- ✓ 1 3/4 lbs. cod or haddock (wild-caught)

DIRECTIONS:

- ➢ Clean your fish and slice into 1" pieces.
- ➢ Sprinkle with the seasoning
- ➢ Toss over to coat the fish thoroughly.
- ➢ Heat the Olive Oil over medium-high flame in a big, nonstickfrying pan.

- ➢ Add the fish and cook for about 10 to 12 minutes until the fish is transparent
- ➢ Splits into pieces. Be cautious not to overcook; otherwise, the fish may be dry and chewy.
- ➢ With your favorite condiments, serve warm.
- ➢ Makes about 4 servings.

NUTRITION INFORMATION: 748 kcal-Protein: 29.23 g-Fat: 6.64 g Carbohydrates 148.64 g

3 STUFFED SAUSAGE MUSHROOMS

Servings: 4 **Cook Time: 25Min** **Prep Time 10 Min**

INGREDIENTS:

- ✓ 4 large Portobello mushrooms (caps and stems)
- ✓ 1 capful (1 Tablespoon)
- ✓ Garlic & Spring Onion Seasoning or Garlic Gusto Seasoning or chopped garlic
- ✓ Chopped chives, garlic powder
- ✓ Onion powder
- ✓ Salt, and pepper to taste
- ✓ 1 1/2 pounds lean Italian sausage (85-94% lean)

DIRECTIONS:

- ➤ Preheat the oven to 350 ° C
- ➤ Cut the mushroom stems carefully and clean both the tops and stems,
- ➤ The stems are chopped into tiny pieces
- ➤ Placed in a bowl Put the meat and spices to the bowl
- ➤ Mix all the spices well, using your fingertips

- ➤ Set the smooth side of the mushroom caps on a wide cookie sheet or baking tray.
- ➤ Divide 4 equal sections of the meat mixture
- ➤ Lightly press one section into each mushroom head.
- ➤ Bake with your favorite side dishes for about 25 minutes & serve crispy

NUTRITION INFORMATION: 437 kcal-Protein: 31.52 g-Fat: 30.89 g -Carbohydrates:16.74 g

4 SMOKY SHRIMP CHIPOTLE

Servings: 4 **Cook Time: 15Min** **Prep Time 15 Min**

INGREDIENTS:

- ✓ 1 capful (1 Tablespoon)
- ✓ Cinnamon
- ✓ Chipotle or a small amount of chipotle pepper
- ✓ Cinnamon, salt, and pepper to taste
- ✓ Teaspoons Olive Oil
- ✓ Fresh garlic
- ✓ 4 T fresh cilantro (optional)

- ✓ 2 lbs. wild-caught
- ✓ Raw shrimp shelled
- ✓ Deveined & tails removed
- ✓ 1 can (16 oz.) diced tomatoes (unflavored, no sugar added)
- ✓ 1 C chopped chives or scallions (greens only)
- ✓ 4 lime wedges (optional)

DIRECTIONS:

- ➤ Heat oil over medium-high heat in a medium-sized frying pan.
- ➤ Put the scallions and roast, until mildly wilted and glistening,
- ➤ for one minute.
- ➤ Include the shrimp and cook on each side for 1 minute.
- ➤ Add the sauce with the tomatoes and Cinnamon Chipotle
- ➤ Cook an extra 3-5 minutes, stirring regularly

- ➤ (Until the tomatoes are hot and the shrimp is thoroughly cooked and opaque)
- ➤ Be careful not to overcook the shrimp which could become hard and dry
- ➤ If needed, sprinkle with cilantro and spritz with a wedge of lime
- ➤ (or for a beautiful and practical garnish
- ➤ Serve the lime wedge on the plate.
- ➤ Serve it warm.

NUTRITION INFORMATION: 632 kcal--Protein: 44.58 g--Fat: 8.71 g --Carbohydrates:176.33 g

5 ONION-MUSHROOM OMELET

Servings: 2　　　　　　**Cook Time: 10Min**　　　　　　**Prep Time 15 Min**

INGREDIENTS:

- ✓ 4 eggs, beaten
- ✓ 1 cup mushrooms, sliced
- ✓ 2 tsp olive oil, divided

- ✓ 1 garlic clove, minced
- ✓ Salt and black pepper to taste
- ✓ ¼ cup sliced onions

DIRECTIONS:

- ➤ Warm the olive oil in a frying pan over medium heat
- ➤ Place in garlic, mushrooms, and onions
- ➤ Cook for 6 minutes, stirring often
- ➤ Season with salt and pepper

- ➤ Increase the heat
- ➤ Cook for 3 minutes
- ➤ Remove to a plate. In the same pan
- ➤ Then in the eggs and ensure they are evenly spread
- ➤ Top with the veggies. Slice into wedges and serve.

NUTRITION INFORMATION: Calories 203, Fat 13g, Carbs 7g, Protein 13g

6 SCRAMBLED EGGS WITH VEGETABLES

Servings: 4　　　　　　**Cook Time: 15 Min**　　　　　　**Prep Time 15 Min**

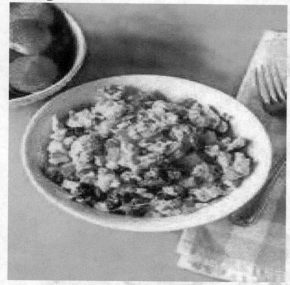

INGREDIENTS:

- ✓ 6 cherry tomatoes, halved
- ✓ 2 tbsp olive oil
- ✓ ½ cup chopped zucchini
- ✓ ½ cup chopped green bell pepper
- ✓ Eggs, beaten 1 shallot, chopped
- ✓ 1 tbsp chopped fresh parsley
- ✓ 1 tbsp chopped fresh basil
- ✓ Salt and black pepper to taste

DIRECTIONS:

- ➤ Warm oil in a pan over medium heat
- ➤ Place in zucchini, salt, black pepper and shallot
- ➤ Cook for 4-5 minutes to sweat the shallot
- ➤ Stir in tomatoes, parsley, and basil
- ➤ Cook for a minute and top with the beaten eggs
- ➤ Lower the heat and cook for 6-7 minutes
- ➤ (Until the eggs are set but not runny)
- ➤ Remove to a platter to serve.

NUTRITION INFORMATION: Calories 205, Fat 15g, Carbs 4g, Protein 12g

7 CITRUS GREEN JUICE

Serving: 1 **Cook Time: 15 Min** **Prep Time 5 Min**

INGREDIENTS:

- ½ grapefruit
- ½ lemon
- 3 cups cavolo nero
- 1 cucumber
- ¼ cup fresh parsley leaves
- ¼ pineapple, cut into wedges
- ½ green apple
- 1 tsp grated fresh ginger

DIRECTIONS:

- In a mixer, place the cavolo nero, parsley
- Add cucumber, pineapple, grapefruit, apple, lemon, and ginger
- Pulse until smooth.
- Serve in a tall glass.

NUTRITION INFORMATION: Calories 255, Fat 0.9g, Carbs 60.2g, Protein 9.5g

8 PANCETTA & EGG BENEDICT WITH ARUGULA

Servings: 2 **Cook Time: 10 Min** **Prep Time 20 Min**

INGREDIENTS:

- 1 English muffin, toasted and halved
- ¼ cup chopped pancetta
- 2 tsp hollandaise sauce
- 1 cup arugula
- Salt and black pepper to taste
- 2 large eggs

DIRECTIONS:

- Place pancetta in a pan over medium heat
- Cook for 5 minutes until crispy. Remove to a bowl
- In the same pan, crack the eggs and season with salt and pepper
- Cook for 4-5 minutes until the whites are set
- Turn the eggs and cook for an additional minute
- Divide pancetta between muffin halves
- Top each with an egg. Spoon the hollandaise sauce on top
- Sprinkle with arugula to serve

NUTRITION INFORMATION: Calories 173, Fat 7g, Carbs 17g, Protein 11g:

9 LOW CARB SLOPPY JOES

Servings: 4 **Cook Time: 25 Min** **Prep Time 5 Min**

INGREDIENTS:

- ½ Tablespoon Cinnamon Chipotle
- Seasoning or ground cinnamon
- Chipotle paste and garlic
- 1 Tablespoon (one Capful)
- Garlic & Spring Onion
- Seasoning or salt, pepper, crushed garlic
- Garlic powder and onion to taste
- 1 Tablespoon yellow mustard
- 1 teaspoon (one packet) powdered stevia
- 2 Tablespoons tomato paste
- 1/2 C diced green bell pepper
- 1 1/2 pounds lean ground beef
- Dash of Desperation
- Salt and Pepper to taste
- 1 Tablespoon of wine vinegar

DIRECTIONS:

- In a frying pan, place the ground beef
- Place it over medium heat on the burner
- When it is frying, split up the larger pieces of beef.
- Cook the meat for about 7 minutes
- Then add the rest of the ingredients (EXCEPT the broth)
- Whisk to mix. Add the water
- Heat up to medium high until combined.
- When the liquid is boiling, reduce the heat to low and let it steam
- (Until the liquid is somewhat reduced)
- Uncovered for around 10-15 minutes.
- Serve warm & have fun!

NUTRITION INFORMATION: 413 kcal--Protein: 46.92 g--Fat: 19.17 g --Carbohydrates:11.08 g

10 BREAKFAST PIZZA WAFFLES

Servings: 2　　　　**Cook Time: 25 Min**　　　　**Prep Time 15 Min**

INGREDIENTS:

- ✓ 4 large Eggs
- ✓ 4 tbsp. Parmesan Cheese
- ✓ 3 tbsp. Almond Flour
- ✓ 1 tbsp. Psyllium Husk Powder
- ✓ 1 tbsp. Bacon Grease(or Butter)
- ✓ 1 tsp. Baking Powder
- ✓ 1 tsp. Italian Seasoning(or spices of choice)
- ✓ Salt and Pepper to Taste
- ✓ 1/2 cup Tomato Sauce
- ✓ 3 oz. Cheddar Cheese
- ✓ 14 slices Pepperoni (optional)

DIRECTIONS:

- ➤ Add all ingredients (except for tomato sauce and cheese) to a container.
- ➤ Use an immersion blender to blend everything.
- ➤ About 30-45 seconds until the mixture thickens.
- ➤ Heat your waffle iron and add half of the mixture to the waffle iron.
- ➤ Let cook until there is little steam coming out of the waffle iron
- ➤ Once done, remove from the iron
- ➤ Repeat with the second half of the mixture
- ➤ Add tomato sauce (1/4 cup per waffle), and cheese (5 oz. per waffle) on the top of each waffle
- ➤ Then, broil for 3-5 minutes in the oven.
- ➤ Optionally add pepperoni to the top of these
- ➤ Once the cheese is melted and starting to crisp on top
- ➤ Remove it from the oven and serve.

NUTRITION INFORMATION: 526 Calories, 45g Fats, 5g Net Carbs, and 29g Protein

11 BREAKFAST BURGER

Servings: 2　　　　**Cook Time: 40 Min**　　　　**Prep Time 20 Min**

INGREDIENTS:

- ✓ 4 oz. Sausage
- ✓ (2 oz. per serving)
- ✓ 2 oz. Pepper Jack Cheese 4 slices Bacon
- ✓ 2 large Eggs
- ✓ 1 tbsp. Butter
- ✓ 1 tbsp. PB Fit Powder Salt and Pepper to Taste

DIRECTIONS:

- ➤ Start by cooking the bacon
- ➤ Lay the strips (however many you want) on a wire rack over a cookie sheet
- ➤ Bake at 400F for 20-25 minutes or until crisp.
- ➤ Mix butter and PB Fit powder in a small container to re-hydrate.
- ➤ Set aside.
- ➤ Form the sausage patties
- ➤ Cook them in a pan over medium-high heat.
- ➤ Flip when the bottom side is browned.
- ➤ Grate the cheese and have it ready.
- ➤ Once the other side of the sausage patty is browned
- ➤ Add cheese and cover with a cloche or lid.
- ➤ Remove sausage patties with melted cheese and set aside
- ➤ Fry an egg over easy in the same pan.
- ➤ Assemble everything: sausage patty, egg, bacon, and rehydrated

NUTRITION INFORMATION: 655 Calories, 56g Fats, 3g Net Carbs, and 30.5g Protein.

12 TEX-MEX SEARED SALMON

Servings: 4   **Cook Time: 15 Min**   **Prep Time 5 Min**

INGREDIENTS:

- ✓ 1 Tablespoon (one Capful)
- ✓ Phoenix Sunrise Seasoning or salt, pepper
- ✓ Garlic
- ✓ Cumin
- ✓ Paprika
- ✓ Cayenne, and onion to taste
- ✓ 1 1/2 pounds wild-caught salmon filet (will cook best if you have it at room temp)

DIRECTIONS:

- ➤ Preheat a nonstick pan for 1 min over high heat
- ➤ Swirl seasoning over the salmon during the heating process (NOT on the skin side)
- ➤ Decrease the heat to medium height.
- ➤ Put the fish in the pan and let it cook for about 4-6 minutes depending on the size, seasoned side down
- ➤ When a "crust" has been created from the seasoning and the fish is quickly released from the pan, you will know it's ready to flip.
- ➤ Lower the heat to medium-low
- ➤ Turn the fish down to the side of the skin
- ➤ Cook for about 4-6 more minutes
- ➤ (Less for medium / rare and more for well done)
- ➤ Using a meat thermometer is the safest way to search for crispiness.
- ➤ We cook to 130 degrees
- ➤ Then let it rest for 5 minutes, not overcooked and softly yellow.
- ➤ Withdraw from the flame and serve
- ➤ Fish can slip on to the plate right off the skin

NUTRITION INFORMATION: 244 kcal--Protein: 42.94 g--Fat: 7.91 g Carbohydrates:0.23 g

13 CHILI ZUCCHINI & EGG NESTS

Servings: 4   **Cook Time: 15 Min**   **Prep Time 25 Min**

INGREDIENTS:

- ✓ 4 eggs
- ✓ 2 tbsp olive oil
- ✓ 1 lb zucchinis, shredded
- ✓ Salt and black pepper to taste
- ✓ ½ red chili pepper, seeded
- ✓ Minced 2 tbsp parsley, chopped

DIRECTIONS:

- ➤ Preheat the oven to 360 F
- ➤ Combine zucchini, salt, pepper, and *olive oil in a bowl*
- ➤ Form nest shapes with a spoon onto a greased baking sheet
- ➤ Crack an egg into each nest and season with salt, pepper, and chili pepper
- ➤ Bake for 11 minutes
- ➤ Serve topped with parsley.

NUTRITION INFORMATION: Calories 141, Fat 11.6g, Carbs 4.2g, Protein 7g

14 CHARRED SIRLOIN WITH CREAMY HORSERADISH SAUCE

Servings: 4　　　　　**Cook Time: 15 Min**　　　　　**Prep Time 5 Min**

INGREDIENTS:

- ✓ 1-3 T horseradish (from the jar)
- ✓ 6 Tablespoons low-fat sour cream
- ✓ 1/2 capful
- ✓ (1/2 Tablespoon)
- ✓ Dash of seasoning or salt, pepper, garlic, and onion to taste
- ✓ 1 1/2 pounds sirloin steaks, trimmed & visible fat removed

DIRECTIONS:

- ➤ Preheat the grill to a medium-high temperature.
- ➤ On all sides, season the steak with Splash of Despair Seasoning.
- ➤ Put on the grill and cook on either side for about 5-7 minutes
- ➤ (Based on how thin the steak is and how fried you like your beef)
- ➤ For rare, you'll leave it on less and for medium-well on more.
- ➤ Use a meat thermometer is the perfect way to prepare your steak.
- ➤ When the meat is cooked, mix the sour cream and horseradish to make the sauce
- ➤ To thin the mixture to produce a sauce
- ➤ Add water, one teaspoon at a time. Put aside until done.
- ➤ Let it sit for five min on a cutting board when the meat is done frying, then slice thinly.

NUTRITION INFORMATION: 370 kcal--Protein: 37.03 g--Fat: 22.42 g --Carbohydrates:2.68 g

15 LOW CARB TACO BOWLS

Servings: 4　　　　　Cook Time: 20 Min　　　　　Prep Time 5 Min

INGREDIENTS:

- ✓ Cauliflower rice
- ✓ 1 large head cauliflower, steamed until soft or frozen ready-to- cook
- ✓ 1 1/2 pounds lean ground beef
- ✓ 2 canned, diced tomatoes (no sugar added, no flavor added)
- ✓ 1-2 capfuls Sunrise or Southwestern Seasoning or low salt taco seasoning

DIRECTIONS:

- ➤ Over medium-high heat, position a large frying pan.
- ➤ In a wide (preferably Nonstick) skillet
- ➤ Add ground beef and sauté for 8- 12 minutes until lightly browned
- ➤ Using a spatula or a cutting implement
- ➤ Cut the bigger bits into smaller parts.
- ➤ Then the tomatoes, then season. Stir to blend.
- ➤ Reduce the heat to low and allow the mixture to simmer
- ➤ (Until the liquid is reduced by 1/2 and pleasant & solid for 5 minutes)
- ➤ Use a food processor or chopping instrument to chop steamed cauliflower into rice-sized bits while cooking
- ➤ Prepare it according to box Directions for using ready-to-cook cauli rice.
- ➤ In a cup, add 1/2 C of cauliflower rice
- ➤ Finish with 1/4 of the meat mixture
- ➤ Top with your favorite condiments and serve sweet.

NUTRITION INFORMATION: 420 kcal-Protein: 46.54 g-Fat: 19.06 g -Carbohydrates:12.24 g

16 TURK ANDSURF BURGERS

Servings: 4 **Cook Time: 20 Min** **Prep Time 5 Min**

INGREDIENTS:

- ✓ 1 Tablespoon Skinny Scampi
- ✓ Seasoning or garlic, lemon, parsley, onion, salt, pepper, and celery

- ✓ 8 medium raw shrimp, peeled, deveined, and tails removed (each shrimp should be about 1 oz. each)
- ✓ 1 1/4 pounds (20 oz.) ground turkey

DIRECTIONS:

- ➤ Preheat the 350-degree outdoor bbq.
- ➤ Place the turkey in a large bowl
- ➤ Sprinkle with seasoning and blend well with your hands.
- ➤ Shape the turkey mixture into four different patties.
- ➤ Push two raw shrimps in a heart shape softly into the top of the burger.

- ➤ Place on the grill and cook on both sides for 5-7 minutes until finished
- ➤ (An internal temperature of 165 degrees F is required for Turkey)
- ➤ Remove and enjoy with a fantastic side dish from the barbecue!

NUTRITION INFORMATION: 220 kcal-Protein: 29.54 g-Fat: 11.01 g -Carbohydrates:0.45 g

17 GREEK STUFFED MUSHROOMS WITH FETA

Servings: 4 **Cook Time: 30 Min** **Prep Time 10 Min**

INGREDIENTS:

- ✓ Four Portobello mushroom caps (about 4" diameter each) 1/2 C crumbled feta cheese
- ✓ 1/4 teaspoon Dash of Desperation Seasoning (or sea salt and fresh cracked pepper)

- ✓ 1 Tablespoon Mediterranean Seasoning (or basil, oregano, onion, black pepper, rosemary, sage, and parsley)
- ✓ 1 1/2 pounds lean ground beef (or chicken, turkey, or lamb)

DIRECTIONS:

- ➤ In a large dish, combine the meat, seasonings, and feta together
- ➤ Gently blend the mixture with both fingertips
- ➤ Split it into four balls of the same size and leave them in the bowl.
- ➤ In a baking dish, put the mushroom caps (season with a pinch of Desperation's Dash)
- ➤ In a mushroom cap, put a part of the meat mixture

- ➤ Press softly, using your fingertips, so that the mixture fills the cap
- ➤ Repeat the mechanism.
- ➤ Place the baking dish in the oven and cook for 25-30 minutes
- ➤ (Or until the meat's ideal temperature is achieved)
- ➤ Serve warm.

NUTRITION INFORMATION: 411 kcal-Protein: 48.08 g-Fat: 22.54 g -Carbohydrates:0.8 g

18 JALAPENO CHEDDAR WAFFLES

Servings: 2 **Cook Time: 10 Min** **Prep Time 10 Min**

INGREDIENTS:

- ✓ 3 OZ. Cream Cheese
- ✓ 3 large Eggs
- ✓ 1 tbsp. Coconut Flour
- ✓ 1 tsp. Psyllium Husk Powder

- ✓ 1 tsp. Baking Powder
- ✓ 1 oz. Cheddar Cheese
- ✓ 1 small Jalapeno
- ✓ Salt and Pepper to Taste

DIRECTIONS:

- ➤ Mix all ingredients except for the cheese and jalapeno using an immersion blender.
- ➤ Once the ingredients are mixed well and smooth, add cheese and jalapeno.

- ➤ Use an immersion blender again to make sure that all of the ingredients are mixed well.
- ➤ Heat your waffle iron, and then pour on the waffle mix. It took about 5-6 minutes in total
- ➤ Top with your favorite toppings, and serve!

NUTRITION INFORMATION: 338 Calories, 28g Fats, 3g Net Carbs, and 16g Protein

19 HAM AND CHEESE STROMBOLI

Servings: 4 **Cook Time: 35 Min** **Prep Time 10 Min**

INGREDIENTS:
- ✓ 1 1/4 cups Mozzarella Cheese, shredded
- ✓ 4 tbsp. Almond Flour
- ✓ 3 tbsp. Coconut Flour
- ✓ 1 large Egg
- ✓ 1 tsp. Italian Seasoning
- ✓ 4 oz. Ham
- ✓ 5 oz. Cheddar Cheese
- ✓ Salt and Pepper to Taste

DIRECTIONS:
- ➢ Preheat your oven to 400F and in a microwave or toaster oven, melt your
- ➢ Mozzarella cheese. About 1 minute in the microwave, and 10- second intervals afterward
- ➢ (Or about 10 minutes in an oven), stirring occasionally.
- ➢ Combine almond and coconut flour, as well as your seasonings in a mixing bowl
- ➢ Use salt, pepper, and an Italian blend seasoning.
- ➢ When the mozzarella is melted, place that into your flour mixture and begin working it in.
- ➢ After about a minute, when the cheese has had a chance to cool down
- ➢ Add in your egg and combine everything. It helps to use two utensils here.
- ➢ When everything is combined and you've got a moist dough transfer it to a flat surface with some parchment paper.
- ➢ Lay the second sheet of parchment paper over the dough ball
- ➢ Use a rolling pin or your hand to flatten it out.
- ➢ Use a pizza cutter or knife to cut diagonal lines beginning from the edges of the dough to the center
- ➢ Leave a row of dough untouched about 4 inches wide.
- ➢ Alternate laying ham and cheddar on that uncut stretch of dough.
- ➢ Then lift one section of dough at a time and lay it over the top, covering your filling.
- ➢ Bake it for about 15-20 minutes until you see it has turned a golden brown color.
- ➢ Slice it up and serve!

NUTRITION INFORMATION: 306 Calories, 28g Fats, 7g Net Carbs, and 26g Protein.

20 GRILLED SHRIMP SCAMPI

Servings: 4 **Cook Time: 20 Min** **Prep Time 10 Min**

INGREDIENTS:
- ✓ 4 teaspoons Olive Oil
- ✓ 1 3/4 lbs. wild-caught large shrimp, shells removed
- ✓ 1/2 Tablespoons Simply Brilliant Seasoning

DIRECTIONS:
- ➢ In a large pot, add all the ingredients and toss to cover. Let the grill sit until it heats up.
- ➢ Preheat grill to medium-high (about 350 degrees). In a barbecue basket, add the shrimp and put on the barbecue.
- ➢ Cook for 15-20 minutes, tossing it with tongs sometimes
- ➢ When they are dark pink and opaque, you'll know they're thoroughly cooked.
- ➢ Serve chilled or hot.

NUTRITION INFORMATION: 722 kcal-33%-Protein: 29.28 g-Fat: 3.27 g-Carbohydrates: 149.26 g

21 PROTEIN OATCAKES

Serving: 1 **Cook Time: 5 Min** **Prep Time 10 Min**

INGREDIENTS:
- ✓ 70g oatmeal
- ✓ 15g protein 1 egg white
- ✓ 1/2 cup water
- ✓ 1/2 teaspoon cinnamon
- ✓ 60g curd
- ✓ 1 teaspoon cacao powder
- ✓ 15g sugar

DIRECTIONS
- ➤ Mix the oatmeal, protein, egg white, and water in a bowl.
- ➤ Preheat a saucepan to medium heat.
- ➤ Place the mixture into the saucepan.
- ➤ While waiting, prepare the topping by mixing the curd, cinnamon, and sugar in a second bowl.
- ➤ Remove the oatcake from the saucepan when it becomes golden-brown.
- ➤ Serve on a plate.
- ➤ Add the topping and cocoa powder

NUTRITION INFORMATION: Calories: 440 -Protein: 1.1g -Fiber: 0.8g -Carbohydrates: 6.1g

23 MEDITERRANEAN SALMON

Servings: 4 **Cook Time: 12 Min** **Prep Time 2 Min**

INGREDIENTS:
- ✓ Wild caught salmon - 20 ounces
- ✓ Mediterranean seasoning - 1 tablespoon

DIRECTIONS
- ➤ Grease your pan with nonstick cooking spray and heat over medium-high heat.
- ➤ Meanwhile, season the salmon.
- ➤ With the seasoned side down, place the salmon in the pan and allow it to sear for about 2 minutes.
- ➤ Flip and lower the heat to medium.
- ➤ Cover the pan and cook for extra 6 minutes, or until the salmon is well cooked.
- ➤ Then serve.

NUTRITION INFORMATION: 188 -Fats: 8.8g -Carbs: 0g -Fiber: 0 -Sugar: 0g -Protein: 27.5g

24 CITRUS FLOUNDER

Servings: 4 **Cook Time: 10 Min** **Prep Time 5 Min**

INGREDIENTS:
- ✓ 1 3/4 pounds lounder filets -
- ✓ 4 teaspoons Lemon oil (Olive oil and lemon zest)
- ✓ 1-2 tablespoons Citrus dill seasoning (or use any other seasoning you like)

DIRECTIONS
- ➤ Heat the oil over medium-high heat with a nonstick pan
- ➤ Add the fish fillets and sprinkle over with the seasoning
- ➤ Cook each side of the fillets for about 2 minutes, or until it becomes opaque and flaky.
- ➤ Serve.

NUTRITION INFORMATION: Calories:189 -Fats: 6.5g -Carbs: 0g -Fiber: 0g- Sugar: 0g - Protein: 30.7g

25 LEMON RADISHES

Servings: 4 **Cook Time: 30 Min** **Prep Time 5 Min**

INGREDIENTS:
- ✓ Red radish halves - 4 cup
- ✓ 2 teaspoons of olive oil
- ✓ Citrus dill seasoning - 1/2 tablespoon
- ✓ Freshly squeezed lemon - 1/2 tablespoon

DIRECTIONS
- ➢ Preheat your oven to 350.
- ➢ Trim the radish and cut into half and equal sizes.
- ➢ Add and toss all ingredients in a bowl until well combined.
- ➢ Place the mixture in oven-safe dish and cook/roast for 30 minutes
- ➢ Then serve

NUTRITION INFORMATION: Calories: 39 Fats: 2.4g Carbs: 3.9g Fiber: 1.9g Sugar: 2.2g Protein: 0.8g

26 MAHI MAHI BASIL BUTTER

Servings: 4 **Cook Time: 15Min** **Prep Time 5 Min**

INGREDIENTS:
- ✓ Butter - 4 tablespoons
- ✓ Garlic and spring onion seasoning (or use parsley, chopped garlic, and chives) - 1 tablespoon
- ✓ Fresh basil leaves (chopped) - 2 tablespoons
- ✓ Fresh lemon juice - 1 tablespoon
- ✓ Fresh mahi mahi filets (wild caught, or you can use flaky white fish, thinly sliced chicken, or shrimp) - 2 pounds
- ✓ Seasoning (or use salt, garlic, and pepper)

DIRECTIONS
- ➢ With your sauce pot, melt the butter over low heat.
- ➢ Add the garlic seasoning, lemon, and basil.
- ➢ Stir mixture to combine well and set it aside
- ➢ Keep the mixture warm.
- ➢ Grease your pan with nonstick cooking spray and heat it up over medium high heat.
- ➢ Sprinkle over with the seasoning.
- ➢ Once the pan is heated up
- ➢ Add the fish and cook each side for about 3 minutes
- ➢ (Or until the fish is fully cooked)
- ➢ Remove from the pan and drizzle over with the melted butter.
- ➢ Then serve.

NUTRITION INFORMATION: Calories:269 -Fats: 12.9g -Carbs: 0.1g -Fiber: 0g -Sugar: 0.1g -Protein: 36.3g

27 FISH TACOS

Servings: 4 **Cook Time: 15Min** **Prep Time 15 Min**

INGREDIENTS:
- ✓ Cod (or haddock, wild caught) - 1 3/4 lbs.
- ✓ Taco seasoning (low sodium) - 1 tablespoon
- ✓ Roasted garlic oil (Olive oil and fresh garlic) - 4 teaspoons
- ✓ Preferred taco condiment

DIRECTIONS
- ➢ Pat dry the fish and cut it into 1-inch chunks.
- ➢ Sprinkle over with the seasoning and gently
- ➢ Toss thoroughly to coat completely.
- ➢ Add the oil over a nonstick pan and heat over medium-high heat.
- ➢ Add the fish and cook for additional 12 minutes
- ➢ (Or until the fish breaks apart into flakes and turns opaque)
- ➢ Then serve with the condiments.

NUTRITION INFORMATION: 151 -Fats: 1.3g -Carbs: 0.2g -Fiber: 0.1g -Sugar: 0g -Protein: 32.5g

28 GARLIC SEASONED ZOODLES

Servings: 4　　　　　　**Cook Time: 5Min**　　　　　　**Prep Time 5 Min**

INGREDIENTS:

- ✓ Roasted garlic oil (or any other oil you like) - 1tablespoon
- ✓ Zucchini noodles - 6 cups
- ✓ Garlic and spring onion seasoning
- ✓ (Or use a mixture of fresh chopped garlic, pepper, and salt) - 1/2 tablespoon
- ✓ Pinch of salt and pepper

DIRECTIONS:

- ➤ With your pan, heat the oil over medium-high heat.
- ➤ Add the noodles and sprinkle over with the seasoning.
- ➤ Cook for about 3 minutes. Toss occasionally.
- ➤ Season with a pinch of pepper and salt.
- ➤ Serve.

NUTRITION INFORMATION: Calories:57 -Fats: 3.7g -Carbs: 5.7g -Fiber: 1.9g -Sugar: 2.9g -Protein: 2.1g

29 CAULIFLOWER SCALLOPS

Servings: 4　　　　　　**Cook Time: 25Min**　　　　　　**Prep Time 5 Min**

INGREDIENTS:

- ✓ Dry sea scallops (or use skinless and boneless chicken breasts, 1-inch chunks) - 2 pounds
- ✓ Seasoning (or use salt & pepper) - 1 teaspoon
- ✓ 4 teaspoon Olive Oil
- ✓ Diced tomatoes (no added sugar) - 3 cup
- ✓ Cajun seasoning (or use any blackening seasoning) 2 teaspoons
- ✓ Fresh lime juice - 2 tablespoon
- ✓ Cooked cauliflower rice - 3 cup
- ✓ To garnish, use sliced scallion greens and fresh cilantro

DIRECTIONS:

- ➤ Pat dry the scallops with paper towel
- ➤ Season with pepper and salt.
- ➤ Add the oil to a pan and heat over medium-high heat.
- ➤ Add the scallops to the pan and cook on each side for about 2 minutes, or until they turn brown.
- ➤ For chicken, cook for 7 minutes, or until it turns brown.
- ➤ Remove the scallops and set them aside.
- ➤ Add the seasonings and tomatoes to the pan.
- ➤ Bring mixture to a boil and scrape all the brown bits from the bottom of the pan.
- ➤ Once it starts to boil, lower heat to medium and simmer for about 10 minutes.
- ➤ Return the scallops to the pan
- ➤ Cook for extra 5 minutes, or until it is fully cooked
- ➤ For chicken, allow it to cook for about 15 minutes.
- ➤ Serve.

NUTRITION INFORMATION: Calories: 258 -Fats: 6.4g -Carbs: 13.9g -Fiber: 3.5g-Sugar: 5.4g -Protein: 36g

30 GRILLED MEDITERRANEAN LAMB BURGERS

Servings: 4   **Cook Time: 15Min**   **Prep Time 5 Min**

INGREDIENTS:

- ✓ Ground lamb (you can use other ground meat) - 1 1/4 lbs.
- ✓ Mediterranean seasoning (or use a mixture of basil, oregano, marjoram, onion, garlic, and parsley) - 1 tablespoon
- ✓ Seasoning (or use a mixture of onion, garlic, salt, & pepper) - 1/2 tsp.

DIRECTIONS:

- ➢ Preheat your grill to medium-high heat.
- ➢ Mix all the ingredients in a bowl.
- ➢ Equally divide the mixture into 4 portions.
- ➢ Press the portions into 1/3-inch thick patties.
- ➢ Place the patties on the grill and cook each side for about 5 minutes.
- ➢ Remove from heat and serve.

NUTRITION INFORMATION: Calories: 313 -Fats: 21.7g -Carbs: 0g -Fiber: 0g -Sugar: 0g -Protein: 27.4g

31 MINI PANCAKE DONUTS

Servings: 8   **Cook Time: 25 Min**   **Prep Time 5 Min**

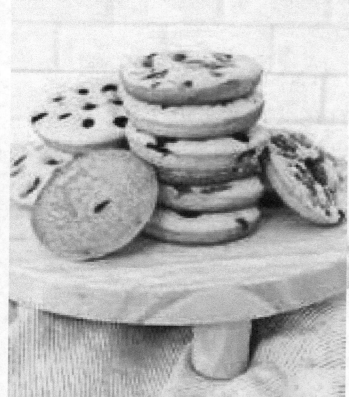

INGREDIENTS:

- ✓ 3 OZ. Cream Cheese 3 large Eggs
- ✓ 4 tbsp. Almond Flour
- ✓ 1 tbsp. Coconut Flour
- ✓ 1 tsp. Baking Powder
- ✓ 1 tsp. Vanilla Extract
- ✓ 4 tbsp. Erythritol
- ✓ 10 drops Liquid Stevia

DIRECTIONS:

- ➢ Stick all of the ingredients inside of a container and mix them using an immersion blender.
- ➢ Make sure that you continue to mix everything for about 45-60 seconds
- ➢ (Ensuring a smooth batter that's slightly thickened)
- ➢ Heat donut maker and spray with coconut oil to ensure non-stick properties
- ➢ Pour batter into each well of the donut maker, filling about 90% of the way.
- ➢ Let cook for 3 minutes on one side
- ➢ Then flip and cook for an additional 2 minutes
- ➢ This is more time than my donut maker tells me to cook them
- ➢ Remove donuts from the donut maker and set them aside to cool
- ➢ Repeat the process with the rest of the batter.
- ➢ This makes a total of 22 Mini Pancake Donuts.

NUTRITION INFORMATION: 32 Calories, 7g Fats, 0.4g Net Carbs, and 4g Protein.

32 WHITE PIZZA WITH BROCCOLI CRUST

Servings: 2   **Cook Time: 35 Min**   **Prep Time 10 Min**

INGREDIENTS:

- ✓ 2 1/2 cups broccoli (riced)
- ✓ 1 egg
- ✓ 1/3 cup + ¾ cup shredded mozzarella cheese (low-fat)
- ✓ 1/4 cup grated Parmesan cheese
- ✓ 1/2 tsp. Italian seasoning
- ✓ 1/2 cup ricotta cheese (part-skim)
- ✓ 1/4 tsp. red pepper flakes
- ✓ 1 garlic clove (minced)
- ✓ 1/2 cup broccoli florets (chopped)

DIRECTIONS:

- ➢ Preheat oven to 400°F.
- ➢ Cook broccoli in a microwave-safe tray and then cover it (about 3 minutes).
- ➢ Once cooled, transfer "rice" to a cheesecloth or clean, thin dishtowel, and squeeze out as much liquid as possible.
- ➢ Take a bowl and mix in broccoli, egg, one-third cup Mozzarella cheese, Parmesan cheese, and Italian seasoning, and combine well.
- ➢ Form mixture into a square pizza (1/3 inch thick) onto a baking sheet. Bake until edges are brown (15-20 minutes).
- ➢ Meanwhile, take a bowl and combine ricotta, red pepper flakes, and garlic
- ➢ Then spread this ricotta mixture onto broccoli crust
- ➢ Sprinkle with the remaining mozzarella, and top with broccoli. Bake for an additional until cheese is melted (about 5-10 minutes).

NUTRITION INFORMATION: 279 kcal-protein:23.85 g-Fat: 16.72 g-Carbohydrates: 9.51 g

33 VEGETABLE EGG BAKE

Servings: 4   **Cook Time: 30 Min**   **Prep Time 10 Min**

INGREDIENTS:

- ✓ ½ cup whole milk 8 eggs
- ✓ 1 cup spinach, chopped
- ✓ 4 oz canned artichokes, chopped
- ✓ 1 garlic clove, minced
- ✓ ½ cup Parmesan cheese, crumbled
- ✓ 1 tsp oregano, dried
- ✓ 1 tsp Jalapeño pepper, minced
- ✓ Salt to taste 2 tsp olive oil

DIRECTIONS:

- ➢ Preheat oven to 360 F
- ➢ Warm the olive oil in a skillet over medium heat
- ➢ Then sauté garlic and spinach for 3 minutes
- ➢ Beat the eggs in a bowl.
- ➢ Stir in artichokes, milk, Parmesan cheese, oregano, jalapeño pepper, and salt
- ➢ Add in spinach mixture and toss to combine
- ➢ Transfer to a greased baking dish and bake for 20 minutes
- ➢ (Until golden and bubbling)
- ➢ Slice into wedges and serve.

NUTRITION INFORMATION: Calories 190, Fat 14g, Carbs 5g, Protein 10g

34 CREAMY MASHED CAULIFLOWER AND GRAVY

Servings: 4   **Cook Time: 20 Min**   **Prep Time 10 Min**

INGREDIENTS:

- ✓ 4 cups cauliflower florets
- ✓ 1/4 cup cream cheese (low-fat, softened)
- ✓ 1 tbsp. butter (unsalted, melted)
- ✓ 1 clove garlic
- ✓ 1 tbsp. rosemary

- ✓ 1/4 tsp. salt
- ✓ 1/4 tsp. black pepper
- ✓ 3 tbsp. gravy mix or mushroom gravy mix
- ✓ ¾ cup cold water

DIRECTIONS:

- ➢ Put water in a pot and let it boil
- ➢ Then, boil cauliflower, until easily pierced with a fork (about 10 minutes)
- ➢ Drain and let it cool slightly.

- ➢ Add the cauliflower and the remaining ingredients into a blender and mix until smooth.
- ➢ Prepare gravy according to package directions

NUTRITION INFORMATION: 90 kcal-Protein: 3.75 g-Fat: 5.76 g -Carbohydrates: 7.51 g

35 AWESOME TUNA SALAD

Servings: 2   **Cook Time: 20 Min**   **Prep Time 10 Min**

INGREDIENTS:

- ✓ ½ iceberg lettuce, torn
- ✓ ¼ endive, chopped
- ✓ 1 tomato, cut into wedges
- ✓ 2 tbsp olive oil
- ✓ 5 oz canned tuna in water, flaked
- ✓ 4 black olives, pitted and sliced
- ✓ 1 tbsp lemon juice
- ✓ Salt and black pepper to taste

DIRECTIONS:

- ➢ In a salad bowl, mix olive oil, lemon juice, salt, and pepper
- ➢ Add in lettuce, endive, and tuna and toss to coat
- ➢ Top with black olives and tomato wedges
- ➢ Serve.

NUTRITION INFORMATION: Calories 260, Fat 18g, Carbs 3g, Protein 11g

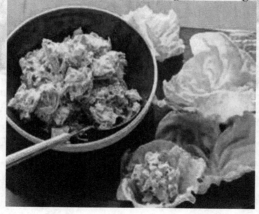

36 ROASTED VEGGIE WITH PEANUT SAUCE

Servings: 4   **Cook Time: 30 Min**   **Prep Time 10 Min**

INGREDIENTS:

- ✓ 1 1/2 cups cauliflower florets
- ✓ 1 1/2 cups broccoli florets
- ✓ 1 1/2 cups red cabbage (cut into bite-sized pieces)
- ✓ 1 bell pepper (remove seeds and membranes, chopped)
- ✓ 1/4 tsp. salt and black pepper (each)

- ✓ 3 1/2 lbs. firm tofu (sliced 1/4 - 1/2 inch blocks)
- ✓ 2 tbsp. peanut butter (powdered)
- ✓ 3 tbsp. water
- ✓ 1/2 tbsp. sambal

DIRECTIONS:

- ➤ Preheat oven to 400°F.
- ➤ Spread all of the vegetables evenly on a lightly greased baking sheet
- ➤ Season with salt and black pepper.
- ➤ Roast veggies until caramelized yet tender
- ➤ Take a pan and sear tofu in a single layer in batches

- ➤ (Until both sides are golden brown)
- ➤ To make a peanut sauce, take a bowl
- ➤ Whisk together the powdered peanut butter, water, and sambal
- ➤ To serve, place tofu in a bowl, top with roasted veggies, and drizzle with peanut sauce

NUTRITION INFORMATION: 623 kcal-Protein: 64.98 g-Fat: 36.3 g -Carbohydrates: 24.08 g

37 SHRIMP & AVOCADO SALAD

Servings: 4   **Cook Time: 15 Min**   **Prep Time 10 Min**

INGREDIENTS:

- ✓ 2 tbsp olive oil
- ✓ 1 tbsp lemon juice
- ✓ 1 yellow bell pepper, sliced
- ✓ 1 Romano lettuce, torn

- ✓ 1 avocado, chopped Salt to taste
- ✓ 1 lb shrimp, peeled and deveined
- ✓ 1 cups cherry tomatoes, halved

DIRECTIONS:

- ➤ Preheat grill pan over high heat
- ➤ Drizzle the shrimp with some olive oil and arrange them on the preheated grill pan
- ➤ Sear for 5 minutes on both sides until pink and cooked through
- ➤ Let cool completely
- ➤ In a serving plate, arrange the lettuce

- ➤ Top with bell pepper, shrimp, avocado, and cherry tomatoes
- ➤ In a bowl, add the lemon juice, salt, and olive oil
- ➤ Whisk to combine
- ➤ Drizzle the dressing over the salad and serve immediately

NUTRITION INFORMATION: Calories 380, Fat 24g, Carbs 23g, Protein 25g

38 CHEESY BROCCOLI BITES

Servings: 4   **Cook Time: 45 Min**   **Prep Time 10 Min**

INGREDIENTS:

- ➤ 6 cups frozen broccoli (steamed-in-bag)
- ➤ 1/4 cup thinly sliced scallions
- ➤ 4 large eggs
- ➤ 2 cups cottage cheese (1%)
- ➤ 1 1/4 cup shredded mozzarella cheese (low-fat)

- ➤ 1/4 cup parmesan cheese
- ➤ 2 tsp. olive oil
- ➤ 1 tsp. garlic powder
- ➤ 1/4 tsp. salt Cooking spray

DIRECTIONS:

- ➤ Preheat oven to 375°F.
- ➤ Cook broccoli according to package directions.
- ➤ Once cooked, add broccoli to the food processor and blend until finely chopped
- ➤ Then, add scallions, eggs, cottage cheese, mozzarella, parmesan, olive oil, garlic

- ➤ Salt to broccoli, and blend until well combined.
- ➤ Scoop mixture into 20 to 24 slots of two lightly greased muffin tins
- ➤ Bake until the filling is set and golden brown (about 25-30 minutes).

NUTRITION INFORMATION: 317 kcal-Protein: 34.05 g-Fat: 13.7 g -Carbohydrates: 18.01 g

39 ONE-PAN EGGPLANT QUINOA

Servings: 4 **Cook Time: 25 Min** **Prep Time 10 Min**

INGREDIENTS:

- ✓ 2 tbsp olive oil
- ✓ 1 shallot, chopped
- ✓ 2 garlic cloves, minced
- ✓ 1 tomato, chopped
- ✓ 1 cup quinoa
- ✓ 1 eggplant, cubed
- ✓ 2 tbsp basil, chopped
- ✓ ¼ cup green olives, pitted and chopped
- ✓ ½ cup feta cheese, crumbled
- ✓ 1 cup canned garbanzo beans, drained and rinsed
- ✓ Salt and black pepper to taste

DIRECTIONS:

- ➢ Warm the olive oil in a skillet over medium heat
- ➢ Sauté garlic, shallot, and eggplant for 4-5 minutes until tender
- ➢ Pour in quinoa and 2 cups of water
- ➢ Season with salt and pepper and bring to a boil
- ➢ Reduce the heat to low and cook for 15 minutes
- ➢ Stir in olives, feta cheese, and garbanzo beans
- ➢ Serve topped with basil.

NUTRITION INFORMATION: Calories 320, Fat 12g, Carbs 45g, Protein 12g

40 CAULIFLOWER LATKES

Servings: 2 **Cook Time: 30 Min** **Prep Time 10 Min**

INGREDIENTS:

- ✓ 2 packets rosemary crackers (ground to a flour-like consistency)
- ✓ 2 1/2 cups cauliflower (riced)
- ✓ 1 egg
- ✓ 1/4 cup onion (diced)
- ✓ 1/4 tsp. salt
- ✓ 1/4 tsp. black pepper
- ✓ Cooking spray
- ✓ 1/2 cup green onion (sliced)
- ✓ 1 cup Greek yogurt (low-fat)

DIRECTIONS:

- ➢ Take a bowl and combine the first six ingredients.
- ➢ Heat a lightly greased pan over medium heat
- ➢ Take one-third of the cauliflower mixture and divided it into two mounds on the pan
- ➢ Flatten each mound into a circular patty (about 1/4 inch thick)
- ➢ Cook them they get a golden brown color (about 3-5 minutes per side)
- ➢ Repeat with the remaining mixture.
- ➢ Garnish with green onions and serve with Greek yogurt.

NUTRITION INFORMATION: 73 kcal-Protein: 4.95 g-Fat: 3.54 g -Carbohydrates: 6.5 g

41 ARUGULA & GORGONZOLA SALAD

Servings: 4 | **Cook Time: 10 Min** | **Prep Time 10 Min**

INGREDIENTS:

- 3 tbsp olive oil
- 1 cucumber, cubed
- 15 oz canned garbanzo beans, drained
- 3 oz black olives, pitted and sliced
- 1 Roma tomato, slivered
- ¼ cup red onion, chopped
- 5 cups arugula Salt to taste
- ½ cup Gorgonzola cheese, crumbled
- 1 tbsp lemon juice
- 2 tbsp parsley, chopped

DIRECTIONS:

- Place the arugula in a salad bowl
- Add in garbanzo beans, cucumber, olives, tomato, and onion and mix to combine
- In another small bowl, whisk the lemon juice, olive oil, and salt
- Drizzle the dressing over the salad
- Sprinkle with gorgonzola cheese to serve.

NUTRITION INFORMATION: Calories 280, Fat 17g, Carbs 25g, Protein 10g

42 GREEK-STYLE PASTA SALAD

Servings: 4 | **Cook Time: 15 Min** | **Prep Time 10 Min**

INGREDIENTS:

- 2 tbsp olive oil
- 16 oz fusilli pasta
- 1 yellow bell pepper, cubed
- 1 green bell pepper, cubed
- Salt and black pepper to taste
- 3 tomatoes, cubed 1 red onion, sliced
- 2 cups feta cheese, crumbled
- ¼ cup lemon juice
- 1 tbsp lemon zest, grated
- 1 cucumber, cubed
- 1 cup Kalamata olives, pitted and sliced

DIRECTIONS:

- Cook the fusilli pasta in boiling salted water until "al dente", 8-10 minutes
- Drain and set asite to cool
- In a bowl, whisk together olive oil, lemon zst, lemon juice, and salt.
- Add in bell peppers, tomatoes, onion, feta cheese
- Then cucumber, olives, and pasta and toss to combine
- Serve immediately.

NUTRITION INFORMATION: Calories 420, Fat 18g, Carbs 50g, Protein 15g

43 ORANGE RICOTTA PANCAKES

Serving: 1   **Cook Time: 5 Min**   **Prep Time 10 Min**

INGREDIENTS:

- ✓ ¾ cup all-purpose flour
- ✓ 1/2 tablespoon baking powder
- ✓ 2 teaspoons sugar
- ✓ 1/2 teaspoon salt
- ✓ 3 separated eggs
- ✓ 1 cup fresh ricotta
- ✓ ¾ cup whole milk
- ✓ 1/2 teaspoon pure vanilla extract
- ✓ 1 large ripe orange

DIRECTIONS:

- ➤ Mix the flour, baking powder, sugar in a large bowl.
- ➤ Add a pinch of salt.
- ➤ In a separate bowl, whisk egg yolk, ricotta, milk, orange zest, and orange juice.
- ➤ Add some vanilla extract for additional flavor.
- ➤ Followed by the dry ingredients to the ricotta mixture and mix adequately.
- ➤ Stir the egg white in a different bowl, and then gently fold it in the ricotta mixture.
- ➤ Preheat saucepan to medium heat and brush with some butter until evenly spread.
- ➤ Use a measuring cup to drop the batter onto the saucepan, ensure the pan is not crowded.
- ➤ Allow cooking for 2 minutes.
- ➤ Flip the food when you notice the edges begin to set, and bubbles form in the center. Cook the meat for another 1 to 2 minutes, serve

NUTRITION INFORMATION: Calories 160 -Fat: 10g -Carbohydrate: 28g -Protein: 6g

44 CHEESY THYME WAFFLES

Servings: 2   **Cook Time: 10 Min**   **Prep Time 15 Min**

INGREDIENTS:

- ✓ ½ cup mozzarella cheese, finely shredded
- ✓ ¼ cup Parmesan cheese ¼ large head cauliflower
- ✓ ½ cup collard greens
- ✓ 1 large egg
- ✓ 1 stalk green onion
- ✓ ½ tablespoon olive oil
- ✓ ½ teaspoon garlic powder
- ✓ ¼ teaspoon salt
- ✓ ½ tablespoon sesame seed
- ✓ 1 teaspoon fresh thyme, chopped
- ✓ ¼ teaspoon ground black pepper

DIRECTIONS:

- ➤ Put cauliflower, collard greens
- ➤ Spring onion and thyme in a food processor and pulse until smooth
- ➤ Dish out the mixture in a bowl and stir in rest of the ingredients
- ➤ Heat a waffle iron and transfer the mixture evenly over the griddle
- ➤ Cook until a waffle is formed and dish out in a serving platter

NUTRITION INFORMATION: Calories: 144 Carbs: 8.5g Fats: 9.4g Proteins: 9.3g Sodium: 435mg Sugar: 3g

45 CHICKPEA AND ZUCCHINI SALAD

Servings: 3   **Cook Time: 0 Min**   **Prep Time 10 Min**

INGREDIENTS:
- ¼ cup balsamic vinegar
- 1/3 cup chopped basil leaves
- 1 tablespoon of capers, drained and chopped
- ½ cup crumbled feta cheese
- 1 can chickpeas, drained
- 1 garlic clove, chopped
- ½ cup Kalamata olives, chopped
- 1/3 cup of olive oil
- ½ cup sweet onion, chopped
- ½ tsp oregano
- 1 pinch of red pepper flakes, crushed
- ¾ cup red bell pepper, chopped
- 1 tablespoon chopped rosemary
- 2 cups of zucchini, diced
- Salt and pepper, to taste

DIRECTIONS:
- Combine the vegetables in a bowl and cover well.
- Serve at room temperature
- But for best results, refrigerate the bowl for a few hours before serving, to allow the flavors to blend.

NUTRITION INFORMATION: Calories:258 Fat:12g Carbohydrates:19g Protein:5.6g Sodium:686mg

46 PROVENCAL ARTICHOKE SALAD

Servings: 3   **Cook Time: 5 Min**   **Prep Time 15 Min**

INGREDIENTS:
- 9 oz artichoke hearts
- 1 teaspoon of chopped basil
- 2 garlic cloves, chopped 1 lemon zest
- 1 tablespoon olives, chopped
- 1 tablespoon of olive oil
- ½ chopped onion
- 1 pinch, ½ teaspoon of salt
- 2 tomatoes, chopped
- 3 tablespoons of water
- ½ glass of white wine
- Salt and pepper, to taste

DIRECTIONS:
- Heat the oil in a skillet. Sauté the onion and garlic
- Cook until the onions are translucent and season with a pinch of salt
- Pour in the white wine and simmer until the wine is reduced by half.
- Add the chopped tomatoes, artichoke hearts and water
- Simmer then add the lemon zest and about ½ teaspoon of salt.
- Cover and cook for about 6 minutes.
- Add the olives and basil. Season well and enjoy!

NUTRITION INFORMATION: Calories:147 Fat:13g Carbohydrates:18g Protein:4g Sodium:689mg

47 BULGARIAN SALAD

Servings: 2 **Cook Time: 20Min** **Prep Time 10 Min**

INGREDIENTS:
- ✓ 2 cups of bulgur
- ✓ 1 tablespoon of butter
- ✓ 1 cucumber, cut into pieces
- ✓ ¼ cup dill
- ✓ ¼ cup black olives, cut in half
- ✓ 1 tablespoon
- ✓ 2 teaspoons of olive oil
- ✓ 4 cups of water
- ✓ 2 teaspoons of red wine vinegar salt, to taste

DIRECTIONS:
- ➤ In a saucepan, toast the bulgur on a mixture of butter and olive oil
- ➤ Leave to cook until the bulgur is golden brown and begins to crack.
- ➤ Add water and season with salt
- ➤ Wrap everything and simmer for about 20 minutes or until the bulgur is tender.
- ➤ In a bowl, mix the cucumber pieces with the olive oil, dill, red wine vinegar and black olives
- ➤ Mix everything well.
- ➤ It combines cucumber and bulgur.

NUTRITION INFORMATION: Calories:386 Fat:14g Carbohydrates:55g Protein:9g Sodium:545mg

48 FALAFEL SALAD BOWL

Servings: 2 **Cook Time: 5 Min** **Prep Time 15 Min**

INGREDIENTS:
- ✓ 1 tablespoon of chili garlic sauce
- ✓ 1 tablespoon of garlic and dill sauce
- ✓ 1 pack of vegetarian falafels
- ✓ 1 box of humus
- ✓ 2 tablespoons of lemon juice
- ✓ 1 tablespoon of pitted kalamata olives
- ✓ 1 tablespoon of extra virgin olive oil
- ✓ ¼ cup onion, diced
- ✓ 2 cups of chopped parsley
- ✓ 2 cups of crisp pita
- ✓ 1 pinch of salt
- ✓ 1 tablespoon of tahini sauce
- ✓ ½ cup diced tomato

DIRECTIONS:
- ➤ Cook the prepared falafels. Put it aside.
- ➤ Prepare the salad. Mix the parsley, onion, tomato, lemon juice, olive oil and salt
- ➤ Throw it all out and put everything aside.
- ➤ Transfer everything to the serving bowls.
- ➤ Add the parsley and cover with humus and falafel.
- ➤ Sprinkle bowl with tahini sauce, chili garlic sauce and dill sauce.
- ➤ Upon serving, add the lemon juice and mix the salad well
- ➤ Serve with pita bread on the side.

NUTRITION INFORMATION: Calories:561 Fat:11g Carbohydrates:60.1g Protein:18.5g Sodium:944mg

49 EASY GREEK SALAD

Servings: 2   **Cook Time: 0 Min**   **Prep Time 15 Min**

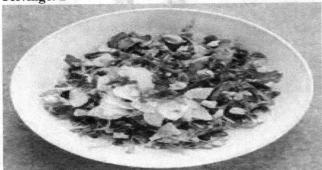

INGREDIENTS:

- ✓ 4 oz Greek feta cheese, cubed
- ✓ 5 cucumbers, cut lengthwise
- ✓ 1 teaspoon of honey
- ✓ 1 lemon, chewed and grated
- ✓ 1 cup kalamata olives, pitted and halved
- ✓ ¼ cup extra virgin olive oil
- ✓ 1 onion, sliced
- ✓ 1 teaspoon of oregano
- ✓ 1 pinch of fresh oregano (for garnish)
- ✓ 12 tomatoes, quartered
- ✓ ¼ cup red wine vinegar salt and pepper, to taste

DIRECTIONS:

- ➤ In a bowl, soak the onions in salted water for 15 minutes.
- ➤ In a large bowl, combine the honey, lemon juice, lemon peel, oregano, salt and pepper.
- ➤ Mix everything.
- ➤ Gradually add the olive oil, beating as you do, until the oil emulsifies
- ➤ Add the olives and tomatoes. Put it right. Add the cucumbers
- ➤ Drain the onions soaked in salted water and add them to the salad mixture
- ➤ Top the salad with fresh oregano and feta
- ➤ Dash with olive oil and season with pepper, to taste.

NUTRITION INFORMATION: Calories:292 Fat:17g Carbohydrates:12g Protein:6g Sodium:743mg

50 ARUGULA SALAD WITH FIGS AND WALNUTS

Servings: 2   **Cook Time: 10 Min**   **Prep Time 15 Min**

INGREDIENTS:

- ✓ 5 oz arugula
- ✓ 1 carrot, scraped
- ✓ 1/8 teaspoon of cayenne pepper
- ✓ 3 oz of goat cheese, crumbled
- ✓ 1 can salt-free chickpeas, drained
- ✓ ½ cup dried figs, cut into wedges
- ✓ 1 teaspoon of honey
- ✓ 3 tablespoons of olive oil
- ✓ 2 teaspoons of balsamic vinegar
- ✓ ½ walnuts cut in half salt, to taste

DIRECTIONS:

- ➤ Preheat the oven to 175 degrees
- ➤ In a baking dish, combine the nuts, 1 tablespoon of olive oil
- ➤ Add cayenne pepper and 1/8 teaspoon of salt
- ➤ Transfer the baking sheet in the oven and bake it until the nuts are golden
- ➤ Set it aside when you are done.
- ➤ In a bowl, incorporate the honey, balsamic vinegar, 2 tablespoons of oil and ¾ teaspoon of salt.
- ➤ In a large bowl, combine the arugula, carrot and figs
- ➤ Then nuts and goat cheese and drizzle with balsamic honey vinaigrette
- ➤ Make sure you cover everything.

NUTRITION INFORMATION: Calories:403 Fat:9g Carbohydrates:35g Protein:13g Sodium:844mg

51 TAHINI VINAIGRETTE WITH CAULIFLOWER SALAD

Servings: 2	Cook Time: 5 Min	Prep Time 10 Min

INGREDIENTS:

- 1 ½ lb. of cauliflower
- ¼ cup of dried cherries
- 3 tablespoons of lemon juice
- 1 tablespoon of fresh mint, chopped
- 1 teaspoon of olive oil
- ½ cup chopped parsley
- 3 tablespoons of roasted salted pistachios, chopped
- ½ teaspoon of salt
- ¼ Cup of shallot, chopped
- 2 tablespoons of tahini

DIRECTIONS:

- Grate the cauliflower in a microwave-safe container
- Add olive oil and ¼ salt. Be sure to cover and season the cauliflower evenly
- Wrap the bowl with plastic wrap and heat it in the microwave for about 3 minutes.
- Put the rice with the cauliflower on a baking sheet
- Let cool for about 10 minutes. Add the lemon juice and the shallots.
- Let it rest to allow the cauliflower to absorb the flavor.
- Add the mixture of tahini, cherries, parsley, mint and salt
- Mix everything well. Sprinkle with roasted pistachios before serving.

NUTRITION INFORMATION: Calories:165 Fat:10g Carbohydrates:20g Protein:6g Sodium:651mg

52 MEDITERRANEAN POTATO SALAD

Servings: 2	Cook Time: 10 Min	Prep Time 15 Min

INGREDIENTS:

- 1 bunch of basil leaves, torn
- 1 garlic clove, crushed
- 1 tablespoon of olive oil
- 1 onion, sliced
- 1 teaspoon of oregano
- 100 g of roasted red pepper. Slices
- 300g potatoes, cut in half
- 1 can of cherry tomatoes
- Salt and pepper, to taste

DIRECTIONS:

Sauté the onions in a saucepan

- Add oregano and garlic. Cook everything for a minute
- Then the pepper and tomatoes. Season well
- Simmer for about 10 minutes. Put that aside.
- In a saucepan, boil the potatoes in salted water
- Cook until tender, about 15 minutes
- Drain well. Mix the potatoes with the sauce and add the basil and olives
- Finally, throw everything away before serving.

NUTRITION INFORMATION: Calories:111 Fat:9g Carbohydrates:16g Protein:3g Sodium:745mg

53 QUINOA AND PISTACHIO SALAD

Servings: 2   **Cook Time: 15 Min**   **Prep Time 10 Min**

INGREDIENTS:

- ✓ ¼ teaspoon of cumin
- ✓ ½ cup of dried currants
- ✓ 1 teaspoon grated lemon zest
- ✓ 2 tablespoons of lemon juice
- ✓ ½ cup green onions, chopped
- ✓ 1 tablespoon of chopped mint
- ✓ 2 tablespoons of extra virgin olive oil
- ✓ ¼ cup chopped parsley
- ✓ ¼ teaspoon ground pepper
- ✓ 1/3 cup pistachios, chopped
- ✓ 1 ¼ cups uncooked quinoa
- ✓ 1 2/3 cup of water

DIRECTIONS:

- ➢ In a saucepan, combine 1 2/3 cups of water, raisins and quinoa.
- ➢ Cook everything until boiling then reduce the heat
- ➢ Simmer everything for about 10 minutes
- ➢ Let the quinoa become frothy. Set it aside for about 5 minutes.
- ➢ In a container, transfer the quinoa mixture
- ➢ Add the nuts, mint, onions and parsley. Mix everything.
- ➢ In separate bowl, incorporate the lemon zest, lemon juice, currants, cumin and oil
- ➢ Beat them together. Mix the dry and wet ingredients.

NUTRITION INFORMATION: Calories:248 Fat:8g Carbohydrates:35g Protein:7g Sodium:914mg

54 CUCUMBER CHICKEN SALAD WITH SPICY PEANUT DRESSING

Servings: 2   **Cook Time: 0 Min**   **Prep Time 15 Min**

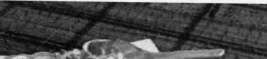

INGREDIENTS:

- ✓ 1/2 cup peanut butter
- ✓ 1 tablespoon sambal oelek (chili paste)
- ✓ 1 tablespoon low-sodium soy sauce
- ✓ 1 teaspoon grilled sesame oil
- ✓ 4 tablespoons of water, or more if necessary
- ✓ 1 cucumber with peeled and cut into thin strips
- ✓ 1 cooked chicken fillet, grated into thin strips
- ✓ 2 tablespoons chopped peanuts

DIRECTIONS:

- ➤ Combine peanut butter, soy sauce, sesame oil, sambal oelek, and water in a bowl.
- ➤ Place the cucumber slices on a dish. Garnish with grated chicken and sprinkle with sauce.
- ➤ Sprinkle the chopped peanuts.

NUTRITION INFORMATION: 720 calories 54 g fat 8.9g carbohydrates 45.9g protein 733mg sodium

55 GERMAN HOT POTATO SALAD

Servings: 12   **Cook Time: 30 Min**   **Prep Time 10 Min**

INGREDIENTS:

- ✓ 9 peeled potatoes
- ✓ 6 slices of bacon
- ✓ 1/8 teaspoon ground black pepper
- ✓ 1/2 teaspoon celery seed
- ✓ 2 tablespoons white sugar
- ✓ 2 teaspoons salt
- ✓ 3/4 cup water
- ✓ 1/3 cup distilled white vinegar
- ✓ 2 tablespoons all-purpose flour
- ✓ 3/4 cup chopped onions

DIRECTIONS:

- ➤ Boil salted water in a large pot
- ➤ Put in the potatoes and cook until soft but still firm, about 30 minutes
- ➤ Drain, let cool and cut finely.
- ➤ Over medium heat, cook bacon in a pan
- ➤ Drain, crumble and set aside. Save the cooking juices.
- ➤ Cook onions in bacon grease until golden brown.
- ➤ Combine flour, sugar, salt, celery seed, and pepper in a small bowl
- ➤ Add sautéed onions and cook
- ➤ Stir until bubbling, and remove from heat.
- ➤ Stir in the water and vinegar
- ➤ Then bring back to the fire and bring to a boil, stirring constantly
- ➤ Boil and stir.
- ➤ Slowly add bacon and potato slices to the vinegar/water mixture
- ➤ Stir gently until the potatoes are warmed up.

NUTRITION INFORMATION: Calories:205 Fat:6.5g Carbohydrates:32.9g Protein:4.3g Sodium:814mg

56 CHICKEN FIESTA SALAD

Servings: 4　　　　　　**Cook Time: 20 Min**　　　　　　**Prep Time 20 Min**

INGREDIENTS:

- ✓ 2 halves of chicken fillet without skin or bones
- ✓ 1 packet of herbs for fajitas, divided
- ✓ 1 tablespoon vegetable oil
- ✓ 1 can black beans, rinsed and drained
- ✓ 1 box of Mexican-style corn
- ✓ 1/2 cup of salsa
- ✓ 1 packet of green salad
- ✓ 1 onion, minced
- ✓ 1 tomato, quartered

DIRECTIONS:

- ➤ Rub the chicken evenly with 1/2 of the herbs for fajitas.
- ➤ Cook the oil in a frying pan over medium heat
- ➤ Cook the chicken for 8 minutes on the side by side or until the juice is clear; put aside.
- ➤ Combine beans, corn, salsa, and other 1/2 fajita spices in a large pan.
- ➤ Heat over medium heat until lukewarm.
- ➤ Prepare the salad by mixing green vegetables, onion, and tomato
- ➤ Cover the chicken salad and dress the beans and corn mixture.

NUTRITION INFORMATION: Calories: 311 Fat:6.4g Carbohydrates:42.2g Protein:23g Sodium:853mg

57 BLACK BEAN & CORN SALAD

Servings: 4　　　　　　**Cook Time: 0 Min**　　　　　　**Prep Time 10 Min**

INGREDIENTS:

- ✓ 2 tablespoons vegetable oil
- ✓ 1/4 cup balsamic vinegar
- ✓ 1/2 teaspoon of salt
- ✓ 1/2 teaspoon of white sugar
- ✓ 1/2 teaspoon ground cumin
- ✓ 1/2 teaspoon ground black pepper
- ✓ 1/2 teaspoon chili powder
- ✓ 3 tablespoons chopped fresh coriander
- ✓ 1 can black beans (15 oz)
- ✓ 1 can of sweetened corn (8.75 oz) drained

DIRECTIONS:

- ➤ Combine balsamic vinegar, oil, salt, sugar, black pepper, cumin and chili powder in a small bowl.
- ➤ Combine black corn and beans in a medium bowl.
- ➤ Mix with vinegar and oil vinaigrette
- ➤ Garnish with coriander. Cover and refrigerate overnight.

NUTRITION INFORMATION: Calories: 214 Fat: 8.4g Carbohydrates: 28.6g Protein: 7.5g Sodium: 415mg

58 AWESOME PASTA SALAD

Servings: 16　　　　　　**Cook Time: 10 Min**　　　　　　**Prep Time 30 Min**

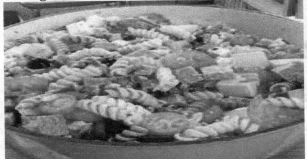

INGREDIENTS:

- ✓ 1 (16-oz) fusilli pasta package
- ✓ 3 cups of cherry tomatoes
- ✓ 1/2 pound of provolone, diced
- ✓ 1/2 pound of sausage, diced
- ✓ 1/4 pound of pepperoni, cut in half
- ✓ 1 large green pepper
- ✓ 1 can of black olives, drained
- ✓ 1 jar of chilis, drained
- ✓ 1 bottle (8 oz) Italian vinaigrette

DIRECTIONS:

- ➤ Boil a lightly salted water in a pot.
- ➤ Stir in the pasta and cook for about 8 to 10 minutes or until al dente
- ➤ Drain and rinse with cold water.
- ➤ Combine pasta with tomatoes, cheese, salami
- ➤ Add also pepperoni, green pepper, olives, and peppers in a large bowl
- ➤ Pour the vinaigrette and mix well.

NUTRITION INFORMATION: Calories: 310 Fat: 17.7g Carbohydrates: 25.9g Protein: 12.9g Sodium: 746mg

59 SOUTHERN POTATO SALAD

Servings: 4　　　　　　　**Cook Time: 15 Min**　　　　　　　**Prep Time 15 Min**

INGREDIENTS:

- ✓ 4 potatoes
- ✓ 4 eggs
- ✓ 1/2 stalk of celery, finely chopped
- ✓ 1/4 cup sweet taste
- ✓ 1 clove of garlic minced
- ✓ 2 tablespoons mustard
- ✓ 1/2 cup mayonnaise
- ✓ Salt and pepper to taste

DIRECTIONS:

- ➢ Boil water in a pot then situate the potatoes
- ➢ Cook until soft but still firm, about 15 minutes; drain and chop
- ➢ Transfer the eggs in a pan and cover with cold water.
- ➢ Boil the water; cover, remove from heat
- ➢ Let the eggs soak in hot water for 10 minutes
- ➢ Remove then shell and chop.
- ➢ Combine potatoes, eggs, celery, sweet sauce
- ➢ Then garlic, mustard, mayonnaise, salt, and pepper in a large bowl
- ➢ Mix and serve hot.

NUTRITION INFORMATION: Calories: 460 Fat: 27.4g Carbohydrates: 44.6g Protein: 11.3g Sodium: 214mg

60 SEVEN-LAYER SALAD

Servings: 10　　　　　　　**Cook Time: 5 Min**　　　　　　　**Prep Time 15 Min**

INGREDIENTS:

- ✓ 1-pound bacon
- ✓ 1 head iceberg lettuce 1 red onion, minced
- ✓ 1 pack of 10 frozen peas, thawed
- ✓ 10 oz grated cheddar cheese
- ✓ 1 cup chopped cauliflower
- ✓ 1 1/4 cup mayo
- ✓ 2 tablespoons white sugar
- ✓ 2/3 cup grated Parmesan cheese

DIRECTIONS:

- ➢ Put the bacon in a huge, shallow frying pan
- ➢ Bake over medium heat until smooth. Crumble and set aside.
- ➢ Situate the chopped lettuce in a large bowl and cover with a layer of an onion, peas, grated cheese, cauliflower, and bacon.
- ➢ Prepare the vinaigrette by mixing the mayo, sugar, and parmesan cheese
- ➢ Pour over the salad and cool to cool.

NUTRITION INFORMATION: Calories: 387 Fat: 32.7g Carbohydrates: 9.9g Protein: 14.5g Sodium: 609mg

61 KALE, QUINOA & AVOCADO SALAD LEMON DIJON VINAIGRETTE

Servings: 4   **Cook Time: 25 Min**   **Prep Time 5 Min**

INGREDIENTS:

- ✓ 2/3 cup of quinoa
- ✓ 1 1/3 cup of water
- ✓ 1 bunch of kale
- ✓ 1/2 avocado, diced and pitted
- ✓ 1/2 cup chopped cucumber
- ✓ 1/3 cup chopped red pepper
- ✓ 2 tablespoons chopped red onion
- ✓ 1 tablespoon of feta crumbled

DIRECTIONS:

- ➤ Boil the quinoa and 1 1/3 cup of water in a pan
- ➤ Adjust heat and simmer until quinoa is tender and water is absorbed for about 15 to 20 minutes
- ➤ Set aside to cool.
- ➤ Place the cabbage in a steam basket over more than an inch of boiling water in a pan
- ➤ Seal the pan with a lid and steam until hot, about 45 seconds
- ➤ Transfer to a large plate
- ➤ Garnish with cabbage, quinoa, avocado, cucumber, pepper, red onion, and feta cheese.
- ➤ Combine olive oil, lemon juice, Dijon mustard, sea salt, and black pepper in a bowl
- ➤ (Until the oil is emulsified in the dressing)
- ➤ Pour over the salad.

NUTRITION INFORMATION: Calories: 342 Fat :20.3g Carbohydrates: 35.4g Protein: 8.9g Sodium: 705mg

62 COBB SALAD

Servings: 6   **Cook Time: 15 Min**   **Prep Time 5 Min**

INGREDIENTS:

- ✓ 6 slices of bacon
- ✓ 3 eggs
- ✓ 1 cup Iceberg lettuce, grated
- ✓ 3 cups cooked minced chicken meat
- ✓ 2 tomatoes, seeded and minced
- ✓ 3/4 cup of blue cheese, crumbled
- ✓ 1 avocado - peeled, pitted and diced
- ✓ 3 green onions, minced
- ✓ 1 bottle (8 oz.) Ranch Vinaigrette

DIRECTIONS:

- ➤ Situate the eggs in a pan and soak them completely with cold water
- ➤ Boil the water. Cover and remove from heat
- ➤ Let the eggs rest in hot water for 10 to 12 minutes
- ➤ Remove from hot water, let cool, peel, and chop
- ➤ Situate the bacon in a big, deep frying pan.
- ➤ Bake over medium heat until smooth. Set aside.
- ➤ Divide the grated lettuce into separate plates
- ➤ Spread chicken, eggs, tomatoes, blue cheese, bacon, avocado
- ➤ Then green onions in rows on lettuce
- ➤ Sprinkle with your favorite vinaigrette and enjoy.

NUTRITION INFORMATION: Calories: 525 Fat: 39.9g Carbohydrates: 10.2g Protein: 31.7g sodium: 701mg

63 MEDITERRANEAN VEGGIE BOWL

Servings: 4   **Cook Time: 20 Min**   **Prep Time 10 Min**

INGREDIENTS:

- ✓ 1 cup quinoa, rinsed
- ✓ 1½ teaspoons salt, divided
- ✓ 2 cups cherry tomatoes, cut in half
- ✓ 1 large bell pepper, cucumber
- ✓ 1 cup Kalamata olives

DIRECTIONS:

- ➤ Using medium pot over medium heat, boil 2 cups of water
- ➤ Add the bulgur (or quinoa) and 1 teaspoon of salt
- ➤ Cover and cook for 15 to 20 minutes.
- ➤ To arrange the veggies in your 4 bowls, visually divide each bowl into 5 sections
- ➤ Place the cooked bulgur in one section
- ➤ Follow with the tomatoes, bell pepper, cucumbers, and olives
- ➤ Scourge ½ cup of lemon juice, olive oil, remaining ½ teaspoon salt, and black pepper.
- ➤ Evenly spoon the dressing over the 4 bowls.
- ➤ Serve immediately or cover and refrigerate for later.

NUTRITION INFORMATION: Calories: 772 Protein: 6g Carbohydrates: 41g

64 ASIAN SCRAMBLED EGG

Serving: 1   **Cook Time: 10 Min**   **Prep Time 10 Min**

INGREDIENTS:

- ✓ 1 large egg
- ✓ 1/2 teaspoons light soy sauce
- ✓ 1/8 teaspoon white pepper
- ✓ 1 tablespoon Olive oil

DIRECTIONS:

- ➤ Beat the eggs in a bowl.
- ➤ To the beaten egg, add soy sauce, one-teaspoon Olive oil, and pepper.
- ➤ Preheat a saucepan on high heat.
- ➤ Add the two tablespoons oil to the saucepan.
- ➤ Then add the mixture of the beaten egg.
- ➤ The edges will begin to cook.
- ➤ Lessen the heat to medium and carefully scramble the eggs.
- ➤ Turn off heat and transfer into a bowl.
- ➤ Serve hot and enjoy

NUTRITION INFORMATION: Calories: 200 Fat: 6.7g Protein: 6.1g Carbohydrates: 1g

65 ARTICHOKE FRITTATAS

Serving: 1   **Cook Time: 30 Min**   **Prep Time 10 Min**

INGREDIENTS:

- ✓ 2.5 oz. dry spinach
- ✓ 1/4 red bell pepper
- ✓ Artichoke (drain the liquid)
- ✓ Green onions
- ✓ Dried tomatoes
- ✓ Two eggs
- ✓ Italian seasoning
- ✓ Salt - Pepper

DIRECTIONS:

- ➤ Preheat oven to medium heat.
- ➤ Brush a bit of oil on the cast-iron skillet.
- ➤ Mix all the vegetables.
- ➤ Add some seasoning.
- ➤ Spread the vegetables evenly in the pan.
- ➤ Whisk the eggs and add some milk.
- ➤ Add some salt and pepper.
- ➤ Mix in some cheese (helps to make it fluffier).
- ➤ Pour the egg mixture in the saucepan.
- ➤ Place the pan inside the oven for about 30 minutes.
- ➤ Enjoy!

NUTRITION INFORMATION: Calories:160 -Protein: 7g -Carbohydrates: 4g -Fat: 3.5g

66 LEAN AND GREEN CHICKEN PESTO PASTA

Serving: 1   **Cook Time: 15 Min**   **Prep Time 5 Min**

INGREDIENTS:

- ✓ 2 cups raw kale leaves
- ✓ 2 tablespoon olive oil
- ✓ 2 cups fresh basil
- ✓ 1/4 teaspoon salt
- ✓ 3 tablespoon lemon juice
- ✓ 3 garlic cloves

- ✓ 2 cups cooked chicken breast
- ✓ 1 cup baby spinach
- ✓ 6 oz. uncooked chicken pasta
- ✓ 3 oz. diced fresh mozzarella
- ✓ Basil leaves or red pepper flakes to garnish

DIRECTIONS:

- ✓ Start by making the pesto, add the kale, lemon juice, basil, garlic cloves, olive oil
- ✓ Then salt to a blender and blend until it is smooth.
- ✓ Add pepper to taste.
- ✓ Cook the pasta and strain off the water
- ✓ Reserve 1/4 cup of the liquid.
- ✓ Get a bowl and mix everything, the cooked pasta, pesto, diced chicken, spinach

- ✓ Add mozzarella, and the reserved pasta liquid.
- ✓ Sprinkle the mixture with additional chopped basil or red paper flakes (optional).
- ✓ Now your salad is ready.
- ✓ Serve it warm or chilled.
- ✓ (Also, it can be taken as a salad mix-ins or as a side dish. Leftovers should be stored in the refrigerator inside an air-tight container for 3–5 days)

NUTRITION INFORMATION: Calories:244 -Protein: 20.5g -Carbohydrates: 22.5g -Fats: 10g

67 MOSTO CARAMELIZED ONIONS

Servings: 10   **Cook Time: 20 Min**   **Prep Time 5 Min**

INGREDIENTS:

- ✓ Onion slices - 1 cup
- ✓ Chicken broth (low sodium) - 1/4 cup
- ✓ Balsamic mosto cotto (or use a balsamic reduction - do not use vinegar) - 4 tablespoon
- ✓ Pinch of sea salt and fresh peppercorns

DIRECTIONS:

- ➢ Add the broth and onions to your pan
- ➢ Cook on a stove over a medium heat for about 20 minutes.
- ➢ Without getting brown, once the onions become soft with the liquid evaporated
- ➢ Add the balsamic to the pan.
- ➢ Turn of the stove and allow the pan on the stove
- ➢ Stir gently and allow the onions to steep into the balsamic.
- ➢ Then serve.
- ➢ It can be stored in a refrigerator for up to 1 week.

NUTRITION INFORMATION: Calories:6 -Fats: 0g -Carbs: 1.4g -Fiber: 0.2g -Sugar: 0.8g -Protein: 0.1g

68 PORK LOIN CARAMELIZED ONIONS

Servings: 4   **Cook Time: 25 Min**   **Prep Time 5 Min**

INGREDIENTS:

➤ Seasoning mix (or use a mixture of any of garlic, black pepper, salt, onion and parsley) - 1 teaspoons

➤ Pork tenderloin (you can use chicken breasts or beef tenderloin)- 1 1/2 lbs.

DIRECTIONS:

➤ Preheat your oven to 400.
➤ Season both sides of the tenderloin.
➤ Over high heat, place the oven-safe pan on your oven
➤ Grease it with nonstick cooking spray.
➤ Once heated up, place the tenderloins in the pan without touching each other.
➤ Cook each side for about 3 minutes, or until it turns brown.

➤ Transfer the tenderloins to the oven
➤ Allow to cook for about
➤ 25 minutes or until well cooked.
➤ Remove from heat and allow it to cool down a bit for about 3 minutes.
➤ Slice the pork.
➤ Meanwhile, prepare the balsamic caramelize onions
➤ Serve with the sliced pork.

NUTRITION INFORMATION: Calories:220 -Fats: 5g -Carbs: 3.8g -Fiber: 0.9g -Sugar: 1.7g -Protein: 37.5g

69 SUNRISE SALMON

Servings: 4   **Cook Time: 15 Min**   **Prep Time 15 Min**

INGREDIENTS:

✓ Wild caught salmon filet (will cook best if you have it at room temp) - 1 1/2 pounds

✓ Sunrise seasoning (or use a mixture of cumin, paprika, salt, cayenne, pepper, garlic, and onion to taste) - 1 tablespoon

DIRECTIONS:

➤ Preheat your nonstick pan for about 1minutesute over high heat.
➤ Meanwhile, sprinkle the seasoning   on the salmon. Don't sprinkle on the skin side.
➤ Low the heat to medium-high heat.
➤ With the seasoned side down, place the salmon on the pan

➤ Cook for about 6 minutes.
➤ Lower the heat further to medium-low and flip the salmon.
➤ Cook for extra 6 minutes.
➤ Serve

NUTRITION INFORMATION: Calories:192 -Fats: 8.8g -Carbs: 0.8g -Fiber: 0g -Sugar: 0.2g -Protein: 27.5g

70 GREEN BEANS GARLIC

Servings: 4   **Cook Time: 10 Min**   **Prep Time 5 Min**

INGREDIENTS:

✓ Green beans (with ends trimmed) - 1 1/2 pounds
✓ Garlic and spring onion seasoning (or use a mixture of pepper, fresh chopped garlic, and salt) - 1/2 tablespoon

✓ Roasted garlic oil (or any other oil you like) - 1tablespoon
✓ Parmesan cheese (freshly grated) - 4 tablespoons

DIRECTIONS:

➤ Add the green beans to a pot.
➤ Add up to 1 inch of water to the pot.
➤ Sprinkle over with the seasoning.
➤ Cover the pot and place it on your stove.
➤ Cook over high heat and bring to boil, about 7 minutes

➤ (Or until the beans steams and becomes crisp tender)
➤ Drain the water and drizzle over with the garlic oil and pepper and salt.
➤ Sprinkle over with the Parmesan cheese.
➤ Serve.

NUTRITION INFORMATION: Calories: 84 -Fats: 5g -Carbs: 7.8g -Fiber: 3.7g -Sugar: 1.5g -Protein: 4g

71 GRILLED LEMON SHRIMP

Servings: 6   **Cook Time: 5 Min**   **Prep Time 20 Min**

INGREDIENTS:

- ✓ 2 tablespoons garlic, minced
- ✓ ½ cup lemon juice
- ✓ 3 tablespoons fresh Italian parsley, finely chopped
- ✓ ¼ cup extra-virgin olive oil
- ✓ 1 teaspoon salt
- ✓ 2 pounds (907 g) jumbo shrimp (21 to 25), peeled and deveined

DIRECTIONS:

- ➢ In a large bowl, mix the garlic, lemon juice, parsley, olive oil, and salt.
- ➢ Add the shrimp to the bowl
- ➢ Toss to make sure all the pieces are coated with the marinade
- ➢ Let the shrimp sit for 15 minutes.
- ➢ Preheat a grill, grill pan, or lightly oiled skillet to high heat
- ➢ While heating, thread about 5 to 6 pieces of shrimp onto each skewer.
- ➢ Place the skewers on the grill, grill pan, or skillet
- ➢ Cook for 2 to 3 minutes on each side
- ➢ (Until cooked through)
- ➢ Serve warm.

NUTRITION INFORMATION: Calories:402 fat: 18g protein: 57g carbs: 4g fiber: 0g sodium: 1224mg

72 ITALIAN FRIED SHRIMP

Servings: 4   **Cook Time: 5 Min**   **Prep Time 10 Min**

INGREDIENTS:

- ✓ 2 large eggs
- ✓ 2 cups seasoned Italian bread crumbs 1 teaspoon salt
- ✓ 1 cup flour
- ✓ 1 pound (454 g) large shrimp (21 to 25), peeled and deveined
- ✓ Extra-virgin olive oil

DIRECTIONS:

- ➢ In a small bowl, beat the eggs with 1 tablespoon water
- ➢ Then transfer to a shallow dish.
- ➢ Add the bread crumbs and salt to a separate shallow dish; mix well.
- ➢ Place the flour into a third shallow dish.
- ➢ Coat the shrimp in the flour, then egg, and finally the bread crumbs
- ➢ Place on a plate and repeat with all of the shrimp.
- ➢ Preheat a skillet over high heat
- ➢ Pour in enough olive oil to coat the bottom of the skillet
- ➢ Cook the shrimp in the hot skillet for 2 to 3 minutes on each side
- ➢ Take the shrimp out and drain on a paper towel. Serve warm.

NUTRITION INFORMATION: Calories: 714 fat: 34g protein: 37g carbs: 63g fiber: 3g sodium: 1727mg

73 COD SAFFRON RICE

Servings: 4   **Cook Time: 35 Min**   **Prep Time 10 Min**

INGREDIENTS:

- ✓ 4 tablespoons extra-virgin olive oil, divided
- ✓ 1 large onion, chopped
- ✓ 3 cod fillets, rinsed and patted dry
- ✓ 4½ cups water
- ✓ 1 teaspoon saffron threads
- ✓ 1½ teaspoons salt
- ✓ 1 teaspoon turmeric
- ✓ Cups long-grain rice, rinsed

DIRECTIONS:

- ➢ In a large pot over medium heat, cook 2 tablespoons of olive oil and the onions for 5 minutes.
- ➢ While the onions are cooking, preheat another large pan over high heat
- ➢ Add the remaining 2 tablespoons of olive oil and the cod fillets
- ➢ Cook the cod for 2 minutes on each side,
- ➢ Then remove from the pan and set aside.
- ➢ Once the onions are done cooking
- ➢ Then the water, saffron, salt, turmeric, and rice, stirring to combine
- ➢ Cover and cook for 12 minutes.
- ➢ Cut the cod up into 1-inch pieces
- ➢ Place the cod pieces in the rice
- ➢ Lightly toss, cover, and cook for another 10 minutes.
- ➢ Once the rice is done cooking, fluff with a fork
- ➢ Cover, and let stand for 5 minutes. Serve warm.

NUTRITION INFORMATION: Calories: 564 fat: 15g protein: 26g carbs: 78g fiber: 2g sodium: 945mg

74 THYME WHOLE ROASTED RED SNAPPER

Servings: 4   **Cook Time: 45 Min**   **Prep Time 5 Min**

INGREDIENTS:

- ✓ 1 (2 to 2½ pounds / 907 g to 1.1 kg) whole red snapper, cleaned and scaled
- ✓ 2 lemons, sliced (about 10 slices)
- ✓ 3 cloves garlic, sliced
- ✓ 4 or 5 sprigs of thyme
- ✓ 3 tablespoons cold salted butter, cut into small cubes, divided (optional)

DIRECTIONS:

- ➢ Preheat the oven to 350°F (180°C).
- ➢ Cut a piece of foil to about the size of your baking sheet
- ➢ Put the foil on the baking sheet.
- ➢ Make a horizontal slice through the belly of the fish to create a pocket.
- ➢ Place 3 slices of lemon on the foil and the fish on top of the lemons.
- ➢ Stuff the fish with the garlic, thyme, 3 lemon slices and butter
- ➢ Reserve 3 pieces of butter.
- ➢ Place the reserved 3 pieces of butter on top of the fish, and 3 or 4 slices of lemon on top of the butter
- ➢ Bring the foil together and seal it to make a pocket around the fish.
- ➢ Put the fish in the oven
- ➢ Bake for 45 minutes
- ➢ Serve with remaining fresh lemon slices.

NUTRITION INFORMATION: Calories: 345 fat: 13g protein: 54g carbs: 12g fiber: 3g sodium: 170mg

75 CILANTRO LEMON SHRIMP

Servings: 4   **Cook Time: 10 Min**   **Prep Time 20 Min**

INGREDIENTS:

- ✓ ⅓ cup lemon juice
- ✓ 4 garlic cloves
- ✓ 1 cup fresh cilantro leaves
- ✓ ½ teaspoon ground coriander
- ✓ 3 tablespoons extra-virgin olive oil
- ✓ 1 teaspoon salt
- ✓ 1½ pounds (680 g) large shrimp (21 to 25), deveined and shells removed

DIRECTIONS:

- ➢ In a food processor, pulse the lemon juice
- ➢ Then garlic, cilantro, coriander, olive oil, and salt 10 times.
- ➢ Put the shrimp in a bowl or plastic zip-top bag
- ➢ Pour in the cilantro marinade, and let sit for 15 minutes.
- ➢ Preheat a skillet on high heat.
- ➢ Put the shrimp and marinade in the skillet
- ➢ Cook the shrimp for 3 minutes on each side. Serve warm.

NUTRITION INFORMATION: Calories: 225 fat: 12g protein: 28g carbs: 5g fiber: 1g sodium: 763mg

76 SEAFOOD RISOTTO

Servings: 4   **Cook Time: 30 Min**   **Prep Time 10 Min**

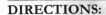

INGREDIENTS:

- ✓ 6 cups vegetable broth
- ✓ 3 tablespoons extra-virgin olive oil
- ✓ 1 large onion, chopped
- ✓ 3 cloves garlic, minced
- ✓ ½ teaspoon saffron threads
- ✓ 1½ cups arborio rice
- ✓ 1½ teaspoons salt
- ✓ 8 ounces (227 g) shrimp (21 to 25), peeled and deveined
- ✓ 8 ounces (227 g) scallops

DIRECTIONS:

- ➢ In a large saucepan over medium heat, bring the broth to a low simmer.
- ➢ In a large skillet over medium heat
- ➢ Cook the olive oil, onion, garlic, and saffron for 3 minutes.
- ➢ Add the rice, salt, and 1 cup of the broth to the skillet
- ➢ Stir the ingredients together
- ➢ Cook over low heat until most of the liquid is absorbed
- ➢ Repeat steps with broth, adding ½ cup of broth at a time
- ➢ Cook until all but ½ cup of the broth is absorbed.
- ➢ Add the shrimp and scallops when you stir in the final ½ cup of broth
- ➢ Cover and let cook for 10 minutes. Serve warm.

NUTRITION INFORMATION: Calories: 460 fat: 12g protein: 24g carbs: 64g fiber: 2g sodium: 2432mg

77 GARLIC SHRIMP BLACK BEAN PASTA

Servings: 4 **Cook Time: 15 Min** **Prep Time 10 Min**

INGREDIENTS:

- ✓ 1 pound (454 g) black bean linguine or spaghetti
- ✓ 1 pound (454 g) fresh shrimp, peeled and deveined
- ✓ 4 tablespoons extra-virgin olive oil
- ✓ 1 onion, finely chopped
- ✓ 3 garlic cloves, minced
- ✓ ¼ cup basil, cut into strips

DIRECTIONS:

- ➤ Bring a large pot of water to a boil and cook the pasta according to the package instructions.
- ➤ In the last 5 minutes of cooking the pasta, add the shrimp to the hot water
- ➤ Allow them to cook for 3 to 5 minutes
- ➤ Once they turn pink, take them out of the hot water,
- ➤ (If they are overcooked, pass them under cold water).
- ➤ Set aside.
- ➤ Reserve 1 cup of the pasta cooking water and drain the noodles
- ➤ In the same pan, heat the oil over medium-high heat and cook the onion and garlic for 7 to 10 minutes. Once the onion is translucent, add the pasta back in and toss well.
- ➤ Plate the pasta, then top with shrimp and garnish with basil.

NUTRITION INFORMATION: Calories: 668 fat: 19g protein: 57g carbs: 73g fiber: 31g sodium: 615mg

78 FAST SEAFOOD PAELLA

Servings: 4 **Cook Time: 20 Min** **Prep Time 20 Min**

INGREDIENTS:

- ✓ ¼ cup plus 1 tablespoon extra-virgin olive oil
- ✓ 1 large onion, finely chopped
- ✓ 2 tomatoes, peeled and chopped
- ✓ 1½ tablespoons garlic powder
- ✓ 1½ cups medium-grain Spanish paella rice or arborio rice
- ✓ 2 carrots, finely diced
- ✓ Salt, to taste
- ✓ 1 tablespoon sweet paprika
- ✓ 8 ounces (227 g) lobster meat or canned crab
- ✓ ½ cup frozen peas
- ✓ 3 cups chicken stock, plus more if needed
- ✓ 1 cup dry white wine
- ✓ 6 jumbo shrimp, unpeeled
- ✓ ⅓ pound (136 g) calamari rings
- ✓ 1 lemon, halved

DIRECTIONS:

- ➤ In a large sauté pan or skillet (16-inch is ideal), heat the oil over medium heat
- ➤ (Until small bubbles start to escape from oil)
- ➤ Add the onion and cook for about 3 minutes, until fragrant
- ➤ Then add tomatoes and garlic powder
- ➤ Cook for 5 to 10 minutes
- ➤ (Until the tomatoes are reduced by half and the consistency is sticky)
- ➤ Stir in the rice, carrots, salt, paprika, lobster, and peas and mix well
- ➤ In a pot or microwave-safe bowl, heat the chicken stock to almost boiling
- ➤ Then add it to the rice mixture. Bring to a simmer, then add the wine.
- ➤ Smooth out the rice in the bottom of the pan
- ➤ Cover and cook on low for 10 minutes, mixing occasionally, to prevent burning.
- ➤ Top the rice with the shrimp, cover
- ➤ Cook for 5 more minutes
- ➤ Add additional broth to the pan if the rice looks dried out.
- ➤ Right before removing the skillet from the heat, add the calamari rings
- ➤ Toss the ingredients frequently
- ➤ In about 2 minutes, the rings will look opaque
- ➤ Remove the pan from the heat immediately
- ➤ (If you don't want the paella to overcook)
- ➤ Squeeze fresh lemon juice over the dish.

NUTRITION INFORMATION: Calories: 632 fat: 20g protein: 34g carbs: 71g fiber: 5g sodium: 920mg

79 CRISPY FRIED SARDINES

Servings: 4   **Cook Time: 5 Min**   **Prep Time 5 Min**

INGREDIENTS:

- ✓ Avocado oil, as needed
- ✓ 1½ pounds (680 g) whole fresh sardines, scales removed
- ✓ 1 teaspoon salt
- ✓ 1 teaspoon freshly ground black pepper
- ✓ 2 cups flour

DIRECTIONS:

- ➢ Preheat a deep skillet over medium heat
- ➢ Pour in enough oil so there is about 1 inch of it in the pan.
- ➢ Season the fish with the salt and pepper.
- ➢ Dredge the fish in the flour so it is completely covered.
- ➢ Slowly drop in 1 fish at a time, making sure not to overcrowd the pan.
- ➢ Cook for about 3 minutes on each side
- ➢ (Or just until the fish begins to brown on all sides)
- ➢ Serve warm.

NUTRITION INFORMATION: Calories: 794 fat: 47g protein: 48g carbs: 44g fiber: 2g sodium: 1441mg

80 ORANGE ROASTED SALMON

Servings: 4   **Cook Time: 25 Min**   **Prep Time 10 Min**

INGREDIENTS:

- ✓ ½ cup extra-virgin olive oil, divided
- ✓ 2 tablespoons balsamic vinegar
- ✓ 2 tablespoons garlic powder, divided
- ✓ 1 tablespoon cumin seeds
- ✓ 1 teaspoon sea salt, divided
- ✓ 1 teaspoon freshly ground black pepper, divided
- ✓ 2 teaspoons smoked paprika
- ✓ 4 (8-ounce / 227-g) salmon fillets, skinless
- ✓ 2 small red onion, thinly sliced
- ✓ ½ cup halved Campari tomatoes
- ✓ 1 small fennel bulb, thinly sliced lengthwise
- ✓ 1 large carrot, thinly sliced
- ✓ 8 medium portobello mushrooms
- ✓ 8 medium radishes, sliced ⅛ inch thick
- ✓ ½ cup dry white wine
- ✓ ½ lime, zested
- ✓ Handful cilantro leaves
- ✓ ½ cup halved pitted Kalamata olives
- ✓ 1 orange, thinly sliced
- ✓ 4 roasted sweet potatoes, cut in wedges lengthwise

DIRECTIONS:

- ➢ Preheat the oven to 375°F (190°C).
- ➢ In a medium bowl, mix 6 tablespoons of olive oil, the balsamic vinegar, 1 tablespoon of garlic powder
- ➢ Then the cumin seeds, ¼ teaspoon of sea salt, ¼ teaspoon of pepper, and the paprika
- ➢ Put the salmon in the bowl and marinate while preparing the vegetables, about 10 minutes.
- ➢ Heat an oven-safe sauté pan or skillet on medium-high heat
- ➢ Sear the top of the salmon for about 2 minutes (Or until lightly brown) Set aside.
- ➢ Add the remaining 2 tablespoons of olive oil to the same skillet
- ➢ Once it's hot, add the onion, tomatoes, fennel, carrot, mushrooms, radishes
- ➢ Join also the remaining 1 teaspoon of garlic powder, ¾ teaspoon of salt, and ¾ teaspoon of pepper
- ➢ Mix well and cook for 5 to 7 minutes, until fragrant. Add wine and mix well.
- ➢ Place the salmon on top of the vegetable mixture, browned-side up
- ➢ Sprinkle the fish with lime zest and cilantro and place the olives around the fish
- ➢ Put orange slices over the fish and cook for about 7 additional minutes
- ➢ While this is baking, add the sliced sweet potato wedges on a baking sheet
- ➢ Bake this alongside the skillet.
- ➢ Remove from the oven, cover the skillet tightly
- ➢ Let rest for about 3 minutes.

NUTRITION INFORMATION: Calories: 841 fat: 41g protein: 59g carbs: 60g fiber: 15g sodium: 908mg

81 LEMON ROSEMARY BRANZINO

Servings: 2 **Cook Time: 30 Min** **Prep Time 15 Min**

INGREDIENTS:

- ✓ 4 tablespoons extra-virgin olive oil, divided
- ✓ 2 (8-ounce / 227-g) branzino fillets, preferably at least 1 inch thick
- ✓ 1 garlic clove, minced
- ✓ 1 bunch scallions, white part only, thinly sliced
- ✓ ½ cup sliced pitted Kalamata or other good-quality black olives
- ✓ 1 large carrot, cut into ¼-inch rounds
- ✓ 10 to 12 small cherry tomatoes, halved
- ✓ ½ cup dry white wine
- ✓ 2 tablespoons paprika
- ✓ 2 teaspoons kosher salt
- ✓ ½ tablespoon ground chili pepper, preferably Turkish or Aleppo
- ✓ 2 rosemary sprigs or 1 tablespoon dried rosemary
- ✓ small lemon, very thinly sliced

DIRECTIONS:

- ➤ Warm a large, oven-safe sauté pan or skillet over high heat until hot, about 2 minutes
- ➤ Carefully add 1 tablespoon of olive oil and heat until it shimmers, 10 to 15 seconds
- ➤ Brown the branzino fillets for 2 minutes, skin-side up
- ➤ Carefully flip the fillets skin-side down
- ➤ Cook for another 2 minutes, until browned. Set aside.
- ➤ Swirl 2 tablespoons of olive oil around the skillet to coat evenly
- ➤ Add the garlic, scallions, kalamata olives, carrot, and tomatoes
- ➤ Let the vegetables sauté for 5 minutes, until softened
- ➤ Add the wine, stirring until all ingredients are well integrated
- ➤ Carefully place the fish over the sauce.
- ➤ Preheat the oven to 450°F (235°C).
- ➤ While the oven is heating, brush the fillets with 1 tablespoon of olive oil
- ➤ Season with paprika, salt, and chili pepper
- ➤ Top each fillet with a rosemary sprig and several slices of lemon
- ➤ Scatter the olives over fish and around the pan.
- ➤ Roast until lemon slices are browned or singed, about 10 minutes

NUTRITION INFORMATION: Calories: 725 fat: 43g protein: 58g carbs: 25g fiber: 10g sodium: 2954mg

82 GRILLED VEGGIE AND HUMMUS WRAP

Servings: 6 **Cook Time: 10 Min** **Prep Time 15 Min**

INGREDIENTS:

- ✓ 1 large eggplant
- ✓ 1 large onion
- ✓ ½ cup extra-virgin olive oil
- ✓ 6 lavash wraps or large pita bread
- ✓ 1 cup Creamy Traditional Hummus

DIRECTIONS:

- ➤ Preheat a grill, large grill pan, or lightly oiled large skillet on medium heat.
- ➤ Slice the eggplant and onion into circles
- ➤ Rub the vegetables with olive oil and sprinkle with salt.
- ➤ Cook the vegetables on both sides, about 3 to 4 minutes each side.
- ➤ To make the wrap, lay the lavash or pita flat
- ➤ Spread about 2 tablespoons of hummus on the wrap.
- ➤ Evenly divide the vegetables among the wraps
- ➤ Lay them along one side of the wrap
- ➤ Gently fold over the side of the wrap with the vegetables
- ➤ Tucking them in and making a tight wrap.
- ➤ Lay the wrap seam side-down and cut in half or thirds.
- ➤ You can also wrap each sandwich with plastic wrap to help it hold its shape and eat it later.

NUTRITION INFORMATION: Calories: 362 Protein: 15g Carbohydrates: 28g

83 ANCHOVY AND ORANGE SALAD

Servings: 4 **Cook Time: 0 Min** **Prep Time 10 Min**

INGREDIENTS:

- ✓ 1 small red onion, sliced into thin rounds
- ✓ 1 tbsp fresh lemon juice
- ✓ 1/8 tsp pepper or more to taste
- ✓ 16 oil cure Kalamata olives
- ✓ 2 tsp finely minced fennel fronds for garnish
- ✓ 3 tbsp extra virgin olive oil
- ✓ 4 small oranges, preferably blood oranges
- ✓ 6 anchovy fillets

DIRECTIONS:

- ✓ With a paring knife, peel oranges including the membrane that surrounds it
- ✓ In a plate, slice oranges into thin circles
- ✓ Allow plate to catch the orange juices
- ✓ On serving plate, arrange orange slices on a layer
- ✓ Sprinkle oranges with onion, followed by olives and then anchovy fillets
- ✓ Drizzle with oil, lemon juice and orange juice
- ✓ Sprinkle with pepper
- ✓ Allow salad to stand for 30 minutes at room temperature to allow the flavors to develop
- ✓ To serve, garnish with fennel fronds and enjoy.

NUTRITION INFORMATION: Calories: 133.9; Protein: 3.2 g; Carbs: 14.3g; Fat: 7.1g

84 SPANAKOPITA DIP

Servings: 2   **Cook Time: 14 Min**   **Prep Time 15 Min**

INGREDIENTS:

- ✓ Olive oil cooking spray
- ✓ 3 tablespoons olive oil, divided
- ✓ 2 tablespoons minced white onion
- ✓ 2 garlic cloves, minced
- ✓ 4 cups fresh spinach
- ✓ 4 ounces (113 g) cream cheese, softened
- ✓ 4 ounces (113 g) feta cheese, divided Zest of
- ✓ 1 lemon
- ✓ ¼ teaspoon ground nutmeg
- ✓ 1 teaspoon dried dill
- ✓ ½ teaspoon salt
- ✓ Pita chips, carrot sticks, or sliced bread for serving (optional)

DIRECTIONS:

- ➤ Preheat the air fryer to 360°F (182°C)
- ➤ Coat the inside of a 6-inch ramekin or baking dish with olive oil cooking spray.
- ➤ In a large skillet over medium heat, heat 1 tablespoon of the olive oil
- ➤ Add the onion, then cook for 1 minute.
- ➤ Then in the garlic and cook, stirring for 1 minute more.
- ➤ Reduce the heat to low and mix in the spinach and water
- ➤ Let this cook for 2 to 3 minutes, or until the spinach has wilted
- ➤ Remove the skillet from the heat.
- ➤ In a medium bowl, combine the cream cheese, 2 ounces of the feta
- ➤ Add the remaining 2 tablespoons of olive oil, along with the lemon zest, nutmeg, dill, and salt
- ➤ Mix until just combined.
- ➤ Join alsoAdd the vegetables to the cheese base and stir until combined
- ➤ Pour the dip mixture into the prepared ramekin
- ➤ Top with the remaining 2 ounces of feta cheese.
- ➤ Place the dip into the air fryer basket and cook for 10 minutes
- ➤ (Or until heated through and bubbling)
- ➤ Serve with pita chips, carrot sticks, or sliced bread

NUTRITION INFORMATION: Calories: 550 fat: 52g protein: 14g carbs: 9g fiber: 2g sodium: 113mg

85 ASIAN PEANUT SAUCE OVER NOODLE SALAD

Servings: 4   **Cook Time: 0 Min**   **Prep Time 10 Min**

INGREDIENTS:

- ✓ 1 cup shredded green cabbage
- ✓ 1 cup shredded red cabbage
- ✓ 1/4 cup chopped
- ✓ Cilantro
- ✓ 1/4 cup chopped peanuts
- ✓ 1/4 cup chopped scallions
- ✓ 4 cups shiritake noodles (drained and rinsed)

ASIAN PEANUT SAUCE INGREDIENTS:

- ✓ ¼ cup sugar free peanut butter
- ✓ ¼ teaspoon cayenne pepper
- ✓ ½ cup filtered water
- ✓ ½ teaspoon kosher salt
- ✓ 1 tablespoon fish sauce (or coconut aminos for vegan)
- ✓ 1 tablespoon granulated erythritol sweetener
- ✓ 1 tablespoon lime juice
- ✓ 1 tablespoon toasted sesame oil
- ✓ 1 tablespoon wheat-free soy sauce
- ✓ 1 teaspoon minced garlic
- ✓ 2 tablespoons minced ginger

DIRECTIONS:

- ➤ In a large salad bowl, combine all noodle salad ingredients
- ➤ Toss well to mix. In a blender
- ➤ Mix all sauce ingredients and pulse until smooth and creamy
- ➤ Pour sauce over the salad and toss well to coat
- ➤ Evenly divide into four equal servings and enjoy.

NUTRITION INFORMATION: Calories: 104; Protein: 7.0g; Carbs: 12.0g; Fat: 16.0g

86 SPANISH GREEN BEANS

Servings: 4 **Cook Time: 20 Min** **Prep Time 10 Min**

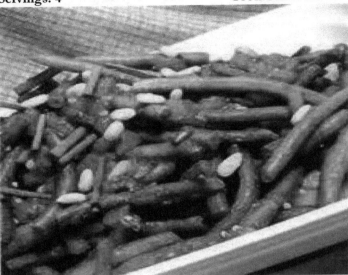

INGREDIENTS:
- ✓ 1 large onion, chopped
- ✓ 4 cloves garlic, finely chopped
- ✓ 1-pound green beans, fresh or frozen, trimmed
- ✓ 1 (15-ounce) can diced tomatoes

DIRECTIONS:
- ➤ In a huge pot over medium heat, cook olive oil, onion, and garlic; cook for 1 minute.
- ➤ Cut the green beans into 2-inch pieces.
- ➤ Add the green beans and 1 teaspoon of salt to the pot and toss everything together
- ➤ Cook for 3 minutes.
- ➤ Add the diced tomatoes, remaining ½ teaspoon of salt, and black pepper to the pot
- ➤ Continue to cook for another 12 minutes, stirring occasionally.
- ➤ Serve warm

NUTRITION INFORMATION: Calories: 200 Protein: 4g Carbohydrates: 18g

87 RUSTIC CAULIFLOWER AND CARROT HASH

Servings: 4 **Cook Time: 10 Min** **Prep Time 10 Min**

INGREDIENTS:
- ✓ 1 large onion, chopped
- ✓ 1 tablespoon garlic, minced
- ✓ 2 cups carrots, diced
- ✓ 4 cups cauliflower pieces, washed
- ✓ ½ teaspoon ground cumin

DIRECTIONS:
- ➤ In a big frying pan on medium heat
- ➤ Heat up 3 tbsps. of olive oil, onion, garlic, and carrots for 3 minutes.
- ➤ Cut the cauliflower into 1-inch or bite-size pieces
- ➤ Add the cauliflower, salt, and cumin to the skillet
- ➤ Toss to combine with the carrots and onions.
- ➤ Cover and cook for 3 minutes.
- ➤ Throw the vegetables and continue to cook uncovered for an additional 3 to 4 minutes.
- ➤ Serve warm.

NUTRITION INFORMATION: Calories: 159 Protein: 3g Carbohydrates: 15g

88 ROASTED CAULIFLOWER AND TOMATOES

Servings: 4　　　　　**Cook Time: 25 Min**　　　　　**Prep Time 5 Min**

INGREDIENTS:

- ✓ 4 cups cauliflower, cut into
- ✓ 1-inch pieces
- ✓ 6 tablespoons extra-virgin olive oil, divided
- ✓ 4 cups cherry tomatoes
- ✓ ½ teaspoon freshly ground black pepper
- ✓ ½ cup grated Parmesan cheese

DIRECTIONS:

- ➤ Preheat the oven to 425°F.
- ➤ Add the cauliflower, 3 tablespoons of olive oil, and ½ teaspoon of salt to a large bowl
- ➤ Toss to evenly coat. Pour onto a baking sheet and spread the cauliflower out in an even layer.
- ➤ In another large bowl, add the tomatoes, remaining 3 tablespoons of olive oil, and ½ teaspoon of salt, and toss to coat evenly
- ➤ Pour onto a different baking sheet.
- ➤ Put the sheet of cauliflower and the sheet of tomatoes in the oven to roast for 17 to 20 minutes
- ➤ (Until the cauliflower is lightly browned and tomatoes are plump)
- ➤ Using a spatula, spoon the cauliflower into a serving dish
- ➤ Top with tomatoes, black pepper, and Parmesan cheese
- ➤ Serve warm.

NUTRITION INFORMATION: Calories: 294 Protein: 9g Carbohydrates: 13g

89 ROASTED ACORN SQUASH

Servings: 6　　　　　**Cook Time: 35 Min**　　　　　**Prep Time 10 Min**

INGREDIENTS:

- ✓ 2 acorn squash, medium to large
- ✓ 2 tablespoons extra-virgin olive oil
- ✓ 5 tablespoons unsalted butter
- ✓ ¼ cup chopped sage leaves
- ✓ 2 tablespoons fresh thyme leaves

DIRECTIONS:

- ➤ Preheat the oven to 400°F.
- ➤ Cut the acorn squash in half lengthwise. Scoop out the seeds and cut it horizontally into ¾-inch-thick slices.
- ➤ In a large bowl, drizzle the squash with the olive oil
- ➤ Sprinkle with salt, and toss together to coat.
- ➤ Lay the acorn squash flat on a baking sheet.
- ➤ Put the baking sheet in the oven and bake the squash for 20 minutes
- ➤ Flip squash over with a spatula and bake for another 15 minutes.
- ➤ Melt the butter in a medium saucepan over medium heat.
- ➤ Add the sage and thyme to the melted butter and let them cook for 30 seconds.
- ➤ Transfer the cooked squash slices to a plate
- ➤ Spoon the butter/herb mixture over the squash
- ➤ Season with salt and black pepper. Serve warm.

NUTRITION INFORMATION: Calories: 188 Protein: 1g Carbohydrates: 16g

90 SAUTÉED GARLIC SPINACH

Servings: 4 **Cook Time: 10 Min** **Prep Time 15 Min**

INGREDIENTS:
- ✓ ¼ cup extra-virgin olive oil
- ✓ 1 large onion, thinly sliced
- ✓ 3 cloves garlic, minced
- ✓ 6 (1-pound) bags of baby spinach, washed
- ✓ 1 lemon, cut into wedges

DIRECTIONS:
- ➤ Cook the olive oil, onion, and garlic in a large skillet for 2 minutes over medium heat.
- ➤ Add one bag of spinach and ½ teaspoon of salt
- ➤ Cover the skillet and let the spinach wilt for 30 seconds
- ➤ Repeat (omitting the salt), adding 1 bag of spinach at a time.
- ➤ Once all the spinach has been added
- ➤ Remove the cover and cook for 3 minutes, letting some of the moisture evaporate.
- ➤ Serve warm with lemon juice over the top

NUTRITION INFORMATION: Calories: 301 Protein: 17g Carbohydrates: 29g

91 CHICKEN BREAST SOUP

Servings: 4 **Cook Time: 4 H** **Prep Time 5 Min**

INGREDIENTS:
- ✓ 3 chicken breasts, skinless, boneless, cubed
- ✓ 2 celery stalks, chopped
- ✓ 2 carrots, chopped
- ✓ 2 tablespoons olive oil 1 red onion, chopped
- ✓ 3 garlic cloves, minced 4 cups chicken stock
- ✓ 1 tablespoon parsley, chopped

DIRECTIONS:
- ➤ In your slow cooker, mix all the ingredients except the parsley
- ➤ Cover and cook on High for 4 hours.
- ➤ Add the parsley, stir, ladle the soup into bowls and serve

NUTRITION INFORMATION: Calories: 445 Fat: 21.1g Fiber: 1.6g Carbs: 7.4g Protein:54.3g

92 CAULIFLOWER CURRY

Servings: 4 **Cook Time: 5 H** **Prep Time 5 Min**

INGREDIENTS:
- ✓ 1 cauliflower head, florets separated
- ✓ 2 carrots, sliced
- ✓ 1 red onion, chopped
- ✓ ¾ cup coconut milk
- ✓ 2 garlic cloves, minced
- ✓ 2 tablespoons curry powder
- ✓ A pinch of salt and black pepper
- ✓ 1 tablespoon red pepper flakes
- ✓ 1 teaspoon garam masala

DIRECTIONS:
- ➤ In your slow cooker, mix all the ingredients.
- ➤ Cover, cook on high for 5 hours, divide into bowls and serve.

NUTRITION INFORMATION: Calories: 160 Fat: 11.5g Fiber: 5.4g Carbs: 14.7g Protein: 3.6g

93 BALELA SALAD FROM THE MIDDLE EAST

Servings: 6   **Cook Time: 0 Min**   **Prep Time 10 Min**

INGREDIENTS:

- ✓ 1 jalapeno, finely chopped (optional)
- ✓ 1/2 green bell pepper, cored and chopped
- ✓ 2 1/2 cups grape tomatoes, slice in halves
- ✓ 1/2 cup sun-dried tomatoes
- ✓ 1/2 cup freshly chopped parsley leaves
- ✓ 1/2 cup freshly chopped mint or basil leaves
- ✓ 1/3 cup pitted Kalamata olives
- ✓ 1/4 cup pitted green olives
- ✓ 3 1/2 cups cooked chickpeas, drained and rinsed
- ✓ 3–5 green onions, both white and green parts, chopped

DRESSING INGREDIENTS:

- ✓ 1 garlic clove, minced
- ✓ 1 tsp ground sumac
- ✓ 1/2 tsp Aleppo pepper
- ✓ 1/4 cup Early Harvest Greek extra virgin olive oil
- ✓ 1/4 to 1/2 tsp crushed red pepper (optional)
- ✓ 2 tbsp lemon juice
- ✓ 2 tbsp white wine vinegar
- ✓ Salt and black pepper, a generous pinch to your taste

DIRECTIONS:

- ➢ Mix together the salad ingredients in a large salad bowl
- ➢ In a separate smaller bowl or jar, mix together the dressing ingredients
- ➢ Drizzle the dressing over the salad and gently toss to coat
- ➢ Set aside for 30 minutes to allow the flavors to mix
- ➢ Serve and enjoy.

NUTRITION INFORMATION: Calories: 257; Carbs: 30.5g; Protein: 8.4g; Fats: 12.6g

94 BLUE CHEESE AND ARUGULA SALAD

Servings: 4   **Cook Time: 0 Min**   **Prep Time 10 Min**

INGREDIENTS:

- ✓ ¼ cup crumbled blue cheese
- ✓ 1 tsp Dijon mustard
- ✓ 1-pint fresh figs, quartered
- ✓ 2 bags arugula
- ✓ 3 tbsp Balsamic Vinegar
- ✓ 3 tbsp olive oil
- ✓ Pepper and salt to taste

DIRECTIONS:

- ➢ Whisk thoroughly together pepper, salt, olive oil
- ➢ Dijon mustard, and balsamic vinegar to make the dressing
- ➢ Set aside in the ref for at least 30 minutes to marinate and allow the spices to combine
- ➢ On four serving plates, evenly arrange arugula
- ➢ Top with blue cheese and figs
- ➢ Drizzle each plate of salad with 1 ½ tbsp of prepared dressing
- ➢ Serve and enjoy.

NUTRITION INFORMATION: Calories: 202; Protein: 2.5g; Carbs: 25.5g; Fat: 10g

95 CHARRED TOMATO AND BROCCOLI SALAD

Servings: 6   **Cook Time: 20 Min**   **Prep Time 10 Min**

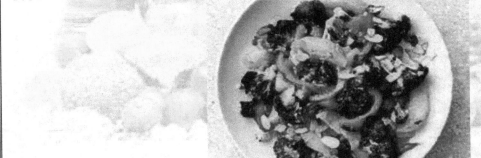

INGREDIENTS:

- ✓ ¼ cup lemon juice
- ✓ ½ tsp chili powder
- ✓ 1 ½ lbs. boneless chicken breast
- ✓ 1 ½ lbs. medium tomato
- ✓ 1 tsp freshly ground pepper
- ✓ 1 tsp salt
- ✓ 4 cups broccoli florets
- ✓ 5 tbsp extra virgin olive oil, divided to
- ✓ 2 and 3 tablespoons

DIRECTIONS:

- ➢ Place the chicken in a skillet and add just enough water to cover the chicken. Bring to a simmer over high heat
- ➢ Reduce the heat once the liquid boils and cook the chicken thoroughly for 12 minutes
- ➢ Once cooked, shred the chicken into bite-sized pieces
- ➢ On a large pot, bring water to a boil and add the broccoli
- ➢ Cook for 5 minutes until slightly tender
- ➢ Drain and rinse the broccoli with cold water. Set aside
- ➢ Core the tomatoes and cut them crosswise
- ➢ Discard the seeds and set the tomatoes cut side down on paper towels
- ➢ Pat them dry. In a heavy skillet, heat the pan over high heat until very hot
- ➢ Brush the cut sides of the tomatoes with olive oil and place them on the pan
- ➢ Cook the tomatoes until the sides are charred. Set aside
- ➢ In the same pan, heat the remaining 3 tablespoon olive oil over medium heat
- ➢ Stir the salt, chili powder and pepper and stir for 45 seconds
- ➢ Pour over the lemon juice and remove the pan from the heat
- ➢ Plate the broccoli, shredded chicken and chili powder mixture dressing.

NUTRITION INFORMATION: Calories: 210.8; Protein: 27.5g; Carbs: 6.3g; Fat: 8.4g

96 ALMOND-CRUSTED SWORDFISH

Servings: 4   **Cook Time: 15 Min**   **Prep Time 25 Min**

INGREDIENTS:

- ½ cup almond flour
- ¼ cup crushed Marcona almonds
- ½ to 1 teaspoon salt, divided
- 1 pounds (907 g) Swordfish, preferably
- 1 inch thick
- 1 large egg, beaten (optional)
- ¼ cup pure apple cider
- ¼ cup extra-virgin olive oil, plus more for frying

- 3 to 4 sprigs flat-leaf parsley, chopped
- 1 lemon, juiced
- 1 tablespoon Spanish paprika
- 5 medium baby portobello mushrooms, chopped (optional)
- 4 or 5 chopped scallions, both green and white parts
- 3 to 4 garlic cloves, peeled
- ¼ cup chopped pitted Kalamata olives

DIRECTIONS:

- On a dinner plate, spread the flour and crushed Marcona almonds and mix in the salt
- Alternately, pour the flour, almonds, and ¼ teaspoon of salt into a large plastic food storage bag
- Add the fish and coat it with the flour mixture
- If a thicker coat is desired, repeat this step after dipping the fish in the egg (if using).
- In a measuring cup, combine the apple cider, ¼ cup of olive oil
- Then parsley, lemon juice, paprika, and ¼ teaspoon of salt
- Mix well and set aside.
- In a large, heavy-bottom sauté pan or skillet
- Pour the olive oil to a depth of ⅛ inch and heat on medium heat

- Once the oil is hot, add the fish and brown for 3 to 5 minutes
- Then turn the fish over and add the mushrooms, scallions, garlic, and olives.
- Cook for an additional 3 minutes
- Once the other side of the fish is brown, remove the fish from the pan and set aside.
- Pour the cider mixture into the skillet and mix well with the vegetables
- Put the fried fish into the skillet on top of the mixture
- Cook with sauce on medium-low heat for 10 minutes
- (Until the fish flakes easily with a fork)
- Carefully remove the fish from the pan and plate
- Spoon the sauce over the fish
- Serve with white rice or home-fried potatoes.

NUTRITION INFORMATION: Calories: 620 fat: 37g protein: 63g carbs: 10g fiber: 5g sodium: 644mg

97 GREEK STYLE QUESADILLAS

Servings: 4   **Cook Time: 10 Min**   **Prep Time 10 Min**

INGREDIENTS:

- 4 whole wheat tortillas
- 1 cup Mozzarella cheese, shredded
- 1 cup fresh spinach, chopped
- 2 tablespoon Greek yogurt

- 1 egg, beaten
- 1/4 cup green olives, sliced
- 1 tablespoon olive oil
- 1/3 cup fresh cilantro, chopped

DIRECTIONS:

- In the bowl, combine together Mozzarella cheese, spinach, yogurt, egg, olives, and cilantro.
- Then pour olive oil in the skillet.
- In the skillet
- Place one tortilla and spread it with Mozzarella mixture.

- Top it with the second tortilla and spread it with cheese mixture again.
- Then place the third tortilla
- Spread it with all remaining cheese mixture.
- Cover it with the last tortilla
- Fry it for 5 minutes from each side over the medium heat.

NUTRITION INFORMATION: Calories: 193 Fat: 7.7g Fiber: 3.2g Carbs: 23.6g Protein: 8.3g

98 LIGHT PAPRIKA MOUSSAKA

Servings: 3 **Cook Time: 45 Min** **Prep Time 15 Min**

INGREDIENTS:

- ✓ 1 eggplant, trimmed 1 cup ground chicken
- ✓ 1/3 cup white onion, diced
- ✓ 3 oz. Cheddar cheese, shredded
- ✓ 1 potato, sliced
- ✓ 1 teaspoon olive oil 1 teaspoon salt
- ✓ 1/2 cup milk
- ✓ 1 tablespoon butter
- ✓ 1 tablespoon ground paprika
- ✓ 1 tablespoon Italian seasoning
- ✓ 1 teaspoon tomato paste

DIRECTIONS:

- ➢ Slice the eggplant in length and sprinkle with salt.
- ➢ In the skillet Pour olive oil and add sliced potato.
- ➢ Roast potato for 2 minutes from each side.
- ➢ Then transfer it in the plate.
- ➢ Put eggplant in the skillet and roast it for 2 minutes from each side too.
- ➢ In the pan Pour milk and bring it to boil.
- ➢ Add tomato paste, Italian   seasoning, paprika, butter,   and Cheddar cheese.
- ➢ Then mix up together onion with ground chicken.
- ➢ Arrange the sliced potato in the casserole in one layer.
- ➢ Then add 1/2 part of all sliced eggplants.
- ➢ Spread the eggplants with 1/2 part of chicken mixture.
- ➢ Then add remaining eggplants.
- ➢ Pour the milk mixture over the eggplants.
- ➢ Bake moussaka for 30 minutes at 355F.

NUTRITION INFORMATION: Calories: 387 Fat: 21.2g Fiber: 8.9g Carbs: 26.3g Protein: 25.4g

99 CUCUMBER BOWL WITH SPICES AND GREEK YOGURT

Servings: 3 **Cook Time: 20 Min** **Prep Time 10 Min**

INGREDIENTS:

- ✓ 4 cucumbers
- ✓ 1/2 teaspoon chili pepper
- ✓ 1/4 cup fresh parsley, chopped
- ✓ ¾ cup fresh dill, chopped
- ✓ 2 tablespoons lemon juice
- ✓ 1/2 teaspoon salt
- ✓ 1/2 teaspoon ground black pepper
- ✓ 1/4 teaspoon sage
- ✓ 1/2 teaspoon dried oregano
- ✓ 1/3 cup Greek yogurt

DIRECTIONS:

- ➢ Make the cucumber dressing: blend the dill and parsley until you get green mash.
- ➢ Then combine together green mash with lemon juice, salt
- ➢ Add ground black pepper, sage, dried oregano, Greek yogurt, and chili pepper.
- ➢ Churn the mixture well.
- ➢ Chop the cucumbers roughly
- ➢ Combine them with cucumber dressing. Mix up well.
- ➢ Refrigerate the cucumber for 20 minutes

NUTRITION INFORMATION: Calories: 114 Fat: 1.6g Fiber: 4.1g Carbs: 23.2g Protein: 7.6g

100 MEDITERRANEAN BURRITO

Servings: 3   **Cook Time: 0 Min**   **Prep Time 10 Min**

INGREDIENTS:

- ✓ 1 wheat tortillas
- ✓ 2 oz. red kidney beans, canned, drained
- ✓ 2 tablespoons hummus
- ✓ 2 teaspoons tahini sauce 1 cucumber
- ✓ 2 lettuce leaves
- ✓ 1 tablespoon lime juice
- ✓ 1 teaspoon olive oil
- ✓ 1/2 teaspoon dried oregano

DIRECTIONS:

- ➤ Mash the red kidney beans until you get a puree.
- ➤ Then spread the wheat tortillas with beans mash from one side.
- ➤ Add hummus and tahini sauce.
- ➤ Cut the cucumber into the wedges and place them over tahini sauce.
- ➤ Then add lettuce leaves.
- ➤ Make the dressing: mix up together olive oil, dried oregano, and lime juice.
- ➤ Drizzle the lettuce leaves with the dressing
- ➤ Wrap the wheat tortillas in the shape of burritos.

NUTRITION INFORMATION: Calories: 288 Fat: 10.2 Fiber: 14.6 Carbs: 38.2 Protein: 12.5

101 SWEET POTATO BACON MASH

Servings: 4   **Cook Time: 20 Min**   **Prep Time 10 Min**

INGREDIENTS:

- ✓ 3 sweet potatoes, peeled
- ✓ 4 oz. bacon, chopped
- ✓ 1 cup chicken stock
- ✓ 1 tablespoon butter
- ✓ 1 teaspoon salt
- ✓ 2 oz. Parmesan, grated

DIRECTIONS:

- ➤ Dice sweet potato and put it in the pan.
- ➤ Add chicken stock and close the lid.
- ➤ Boil the vegetables for until they are soft.
- ➤ After this, drain the chicken stock.
- ➤ Mash the sweet potato with the help of the potato masher
- ➤ Than add grated cheese and butter.
- ➤ Mix up together salt and chopped bacon
- ➤ Fry the mixture until it is crunchy (10-15 minutes).
- ➤ Add cooked bacon in the mashed sweet potato
- ➤ Mix up with the help of the spoon.
- ➤ It is recommended to serve the meal warm or hot.

NUTRITION INFORMATION: Calories: 304 Fat: 18.1 Fiber: 2.9 Carbs: 18.8 Protein: 17

102 PROSCIUTTO WRAPPED MOZZARELLA BALLS

Servings: 4   **Cook Time: 10 Min**   **Prep Time 10 Min**

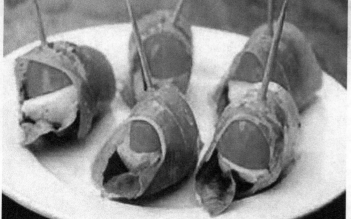

INGREDIENTS:

- ✓ 8 Mozzarella balls, cherry size
- ✓ 4 oz. bacon, sliced
- ✓ 1/4 teaspoon ground black pepper
- ✓ ¾ teaspoon dried rosemary
- ✓ 2 teaspoon olive oil

DIRECTIONS:

- ➤ Sprinkle the sliced bacon with ground black pepper and dried rosemary.
- ➤ Wrap every Mozzarella ball in the sliced bacon and secure them with toothpicks.
- ➤ Brush wrapped Mozzarella balls with oil.
- ➤ Line the baking tray with the parchment and arrange Mozzarella balls in it.
- ➤ Bake the meal for 10 minutes at 365F.

NUTRITION INFORMATION: Calories: 323 Fat: 26.8 Fiber: 0.1 Carbs: 0.6 Protein: 20.6

103 COLESLAW ASIAN STYLE

Servings: 10 **Cook Time: 0 Min** **Prep Time 10 Min**

INGREDIENTS:
- ✓ ½ cup chopped fresh cilantro
- ✓ 1 ½ tbsp minced garlic
- ✓ 2 carrots, julienned
- ✓ 2 cups shredded napa cabbage
- ✓ 2 cups thinly sliced red cabbage
- ✓ 2 red bell peppers, thinly sliced
- ✓ 2 tbsp minced fresh ginger root
- ✓ 3 tbsp brown sugar
- ✓ 3 tbsp soy sauce
- ✓ 5 cups thinly sliced green cabbage
- ✓ 5 tbsp creamy peanut butter
- ✓ 6 green onions, chopped
- ✓ 6 tbsp rice wine vinegar
- ✓ 6 tbsp vegetable oil

DIRECTIONS:
- ➢ Mix thoroughly the following in a medium bowl: garlic, ginger, brown sugar
- ➢ Add soy sauce, peanut butter, oil and rice vinegar
- ➢ In a separate bowl, blend well cilantro, green onions, carrots, bell pepper
- ➢ Then Napa cabbage, red cabbage and green cabbage
- ➢ Pour in the peanut sauce above
- ➢ Toss to mix well
- ➢ Serve and enjoy.

NUTRITION INFORMATION: Calories: 193.8; Protein: 4g; Fat: 12.6g; Carbs: 16.1g

104 CUCUMBER SALAD JAPANESE STYLE

Servings: 5 **Cook Time: 0 Min** **Prep Time 10 Min**

INGREDIENTS:
- ✓ ½ tsp minced fresh ginger root
- ✓ 1 tsp salt
- ✓ 1/3 cup rice vinegar
- ✓ 2 large cucumbers, ribbon cut
- ✓ 4 tsp white sugar

DIRECTIONS:
- ➢ Mix well ginger, salt, sugar and vinegar in a small bowl
- ➢ Add ribbon cut cucumbers and mix well
- ➢ Let stand for at least one hour in the ref before serving.

NUTRITION INFORMATION: Calories: 29; Fat: .2g; Protein: .7g; Carbs: 6.1g

105 GARLIC CHICKEN BALLS

Servings: 4 **Cook Time: 10 Min** **Prep Time 15 Min**

INGREDIENTS:
- ✓ 2 cups ground chicken
- ✓ 1 teaspoon minced garlic
- ✓ 1 teaspoon dried dill
- ✓ 1/3 carrot, grated
- ✓ 1 egg, beaten
- ✓ 1 tablespoon olive oil
- ✓ 1/4 cup coconut flakes
- ✓ 1/2 teaspoon salt

DIRECTIONS:
- ➢ In the mixing bowl mix up together ground chicken, minced garlic, dried dill, carrot, egg, and salt.
- ➢ Stir the chicken mixture with the help of the fingertips until homogenous.
- ➢ Then make medium balls from the mixture.
- ➢ Coat every chicken ball in coconut flakes.
- ➢ Heat up olive oil in the skillet.
- ➢ Add chicken balls and cook them for 3 minutes from each side
- ➢ The cooked chicken balls will have a golden-brown color.

NUTRITION INFORMATION: Calories: 200 Fat: 11.5 Fiber: 0.6 Carbs: 1.7 Protein: 21.9

106 GARLICKY SAUTÉED ZUCCHINI WITH MINT

Servings: 4   **Cook Time: 10 Min**   **Prep Time 5 Min**

INGREDIENTS:

- ✓ 3 large green zucchinis
- ✓ 3 tablespoons extra-virgin olive oil
- ✓ 1 large onion, chopped
- ✓ 3 cloves garlic, minced
- ✓ 1 teaspoon dried mint

DIRECTIONS:

- ➢ Cut the zucchini into ½-inch cubes.
- ➢ Using huge skillet, place over medium heat
- ➢ Cook the olive oil, onions, and garlic for 3 minutes, stirring constantly.
- ➢ Add the zucchini and salt to the skillet
- ➢ Toss to combine with the onions and garlic, cooking for 5 minutes.
- ➢ Add the mint to the skillet, tossing to combine
- ➢ Cook for another 2 minutes. Serve warm.

NUTRITION INFORMATION: Calories: 147 Protein: 4g Carbohydrates: 12g

107 STEWED OKRA

Servings: 4   **Cook Time: 25Min**   **Prep Time 5 Min**

INGREDIENTS:

- ✓ 3 cloves garlic, finely chopped
- ✓ 1 pound fresh or frozen okra, cleaned
- ✓ 1 (15-ounce) can plain tomato sauce
- ✓ 2 cups water
- ✓ ½ cup fresh cilantro, finely chopped

DIRECTIONS:

- ➢ In a big pot at medium heat, stir and cook ¼ cup of olive oil, 1 onion, garlic, and salt for 1 minute.
- ➢ Stir in the okra and cook for 3 minutes.
- ➢ Add the tomato sauce, water, cilantro, and black pepper
- ➢ Stir, cover, and let cook for 15 minutes, stirring occasionally.
- ➢ Serve warm.

NUTRITION INFORMATION: Calories: 201 Protein: 4g Carbohydrates: 18g

108 SWEET VEGGIE-STUFFED PEPPERS

Servings: 6   **Cook Time: 30 Min**   **Prep Time 20 Min**

INGREDIENTS:
- ✓ 6 large bell peppers, different colors
- ✓ 3 cloves garlic, minced
- ✓ 1 carrot, chopped
- ✓ (16-ounce) can garbanzo beans
- ✓ 3 cups cooked rice

DIRECTIONS:
- ➤ Preheat the oven to 350°F.
- ➤ Make sure to choose peppers that can stand upright
- ➤ Cut off the pepper cap and remove the seeds, reserving the cap for later
- ➤ Stand the peppers in a baking dish.
- ➤ In a skillet over medium heat, cook up olive oil, 1 onion, garlic, and carrots for 3 minutes.
- ➤ Stir in the garbanzo beans. Cook for another 3 minutes.
- ➤ Remove the pan from the heat
- ➤ Spoon the cooked ingredients to a large bowl.
- ➤ Add the rice, salt, and pepper; toss to combine.
- ➤ Stuff each pepper to the top and then put the pepper caps back on
- ➤ Cover the baking dish with aluminum foil and bake for 25 minutes.
- ➤ Remove the foil and bake for another 5 minutes.
- ➤ Serve warm.

NUTRITION INFORMATION: Calories: 301 Protein: 8g Carbohydrates: 50g

109 VEGETABLE-STUFFED GRAPE LEAVES

Servings: 7   **Cook Time: 45 Min**   **Prep Time 50 Min**

INGREDIENTS:
- ✓ 1 cups white rice, rinsed
- ✓ 2 large tomatoes, finely diced
- ✓ 1 (16-ounce) jar grape leaves
- ✓ 1 cup lemon juice
- ✓ 4 to 6 cups water

DIRECTIONS:
- ➤ Incorporate rice, tomatoes, 1 onion, 1 green onion, 1 cup of parsley, 3 garlic cloves, salt, and black pepper.
- ➤ Drain and rinse the grape leaves.
- ➤ Prepare a large pot by placing a layer of grape leaves on the bottom
- ➤ Lay each leaf flat and trim off any stems.
- ➤ Place 2 tablespoons of the rice mixture at the base of each leaf
- ➤ Fold over the sides, then roll as tight as possible
- ➤ Place the rolled grape leaves in the pot, lining up each rolled grape leaf
- ➤ Continue to layer in the rolled grape leaves.
- ➤ Gently pour the lemon juice and olive oil over the grape leaves
- ➤ Add enough water to just cover the grape leaves by 1 inch.
- ➤ Lay a heavy plate that is smaller
- ➤ Than the opening of the pot upside down over the grape leaves
- ➤ Cover the pot and cook the leaves over medium-low heat for 45 minutes
- ➤ Let stand for 20 minutes before serving.
- ➤ Serve warm or cold.

NUTRITION INFORMATION: Calories: 532 Protein: 12g Carbohydrates: 80g

110 GRILLED EGGPLANT ROLLS

Servings: 5   **Cook Time: 10 Min**   **Prep Time 30 Min**

INGREDIENTS:

- ✓ 2 large eggplants
- ✓ 4 ounces goat cheese
- ✓ 1 cup ricotta
- ✓ ¼ cup fresh basil, finely chopped

DIRECTIONS:

➤ Slice the tops of the eggplants off and cut the eggplants lengthwise into ¼-inch-thick slices

➤ Sprinkle the slices with the salt and place the eggplant in a colander for 15 to 20 minutes

➤ The salt will draw out excess water from the eggplant.

➤ In a large bowl, combine the goat cheese, ricotta, basil, and pepper

➤ Preheat a grill, grill pan, or lightly oiled skillet on medium heat

➤ Pat the eggplant slices dry using paper towel and lightly spray with olive oil spray

➤ Place the eggplant on the grill, grill pan, or skillet and cook for 3 minutes on each side.

➤ Remove the eggplant from the heat and let cool for 5 minutes.

➤ To roll, lay one eggplant slice flat

➤ Place a tablespoon of the cheese mixture at the base of the slice, and roll up

➤ Serve immediately or chill until serving.

NUTRITION INFORMATION: Calories: 255 Protein: 15g Carbohydrates: 19g

111 CRISPY ZUCCHINI FRITTERS

Servings: 6   **Cook Time: 20 Min**   **Prep Time 15 Min**

INGREDIENTS:

- ✓ 2 large green zucchinis
- ✓ 1 cup flour
- ✓ 1 large egg, beaten
- ✓ ½ cup water
- ✓ 1 teaspoon baking powder

DIRECTIONS:

➤ Grate the zucchini into a large bowl.

➤ Add the 2 tbsps. of parsley, 3 garlic cloves, salt, flour, egg, water

➤ Then baking powder to the bowl and stir to combine.

➤ In a large pot or fryer over medium heat, heat oil to 365°F.

➤ Drop the fritter batter into 3 cups of vegetable oil

➤ Turn the fritters over using a slotted spoon and fry

➤ (Until they are golden brown, about 2 to 3 minutes)

➤ Strain fritters from the oil

➤ Place on a plate lined with paper towels.

➤ Serve warm with Creamy Tzatziki or Creamy Traditional Hummus as a dip.

NUTRITION INFORMATION: Calories: 446 Protein: 5g Carbohydrates: 19g

112 CHEESY SPINACH PIES

Servings: 5   **Cook Time: 40 Min**   **Prep Time 20 Min**

INGREDIENTS:

- ✓ 1 tablespoons extra-virgin olive oil
- ✓ 2 (1-pound) bags of baby spinach, washed
- ✓ 1 cup feta cheese
- ✓ 1 large egg, beaten
- ✓ Puff pastry sheets

DIRECTIONS:

- ➢ Preheat the oven to 375°F.
- ➢ In a frying pan on medium heat, put the olive oil, 1 onion, and 2 garlic cloves for 3 minutes.
- ➢ Add the spinach to the skillet one bag at a time, letting it wilt in between each bag
- ➢ Toss using tongs. Cook for 4 minutes
- ➢ Once the spinach is cooked, drain any excess liquid from the pan.
- ➢ Mix feta cheese, egg, and cooked spinach.
- ➢ Lay the puff pastry flat on a counter
- ➢ Cut the pastry into 3-inch squares.
- ➢ Place a tablespoon of the spinach mixture in the center of a puff-pastry square
- ➢ Fold over one corner of the square to the diagonal corner, forming a triangle
- ➢ Crimp the edges of the pie by pressing down with the tines of a fork to seal them together
- ➢ Repeat until all squares are filled.
- ➢ Situate the pies on a parchment-lined baking sheet
- ➢ Bake for 25 to 30 minutes or until golden brown
- ➢ Serve warm or at room temperature

NUTRITION INFORMATION: Calories: 503 Protein: 16g Carbohydrates: 38g

113 SEA BASS CRUSTED WITH MOROCCAN SPICES

Servings: 4 **Cook Time: 40 Min** **Prep Time 15 Min**

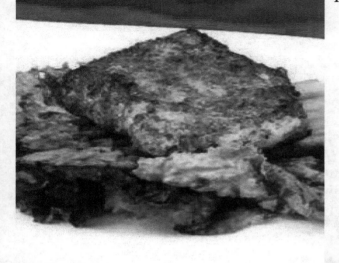

INGREDIENTS:

- ✓ 1½ teaspoons ground turmeric, divided
- ✓ ¾ teaspoon saffron
- ✓ ½ teaspoon ground cumin
- ✓ ¼ teaspoon kosher salt
- ✓ ¼ teaspoon freshly ground black pepper
- ✓ 1½ pounds (680 g) sea bass fillets, about
- ✓ ½ inch thick 8 tablespoons extra-virgin olive oil, divided
- ✓ 8 garlic cloves, divided (4 minced cloves and 4 sliced)
- ✓ 6 medium baby portobello mushrooms, chopped
- ✓ 1 large carrot, sliced on an angle
- ✓ 2 sun-dried tomatoes, thinly sliced (optional)
- ✓ 2 tablespoons tomato paste
- ✓ 1 (15-ounce / 425-g) can chickpeas, drained and rinsed
- ✓ 1½ cups low-sodium vegetable broth
- ✓ ¼ cup white wine
- ✓ 1 tablespoon ground coriander (optional)
- ✓ 1 cup sliced artichoke hearts marinated in olive oil
- ✓ ½ cup pitted Kalamata olives
- ✓ ½ lemon, juiced
- ✓ ½ lemon, cut into thin rounds
- ✓ 4 to 5 rosemary sprigs or
- ✓ 2 tablespoons dried rosemary
- ✓ Fresh cilantro, for garnish

DIRECTIONS:

- ➢ In a small mixing bowl, combine 1 teaspoon turmeric and the saffron and cumin
- ➢ Season with salt and pepper. Season both sides of the fish with the spice mixture
- ➢ Add 3 tablespoons of olive oil
- ➢ Work the fish to make sure it's well coated with the spices and the olive oil.
- ➢ In a large sauté pan or skillet, heat 2 tablespoons of olive oil over medium heat until shimmering but not smoking
- ➢ Sear the top side of the sea bass for about 1 minute, or until golden
- ➢ Remove and set aside.
- ➢ In the same skillet, add the minced garlic and cook very briefly, tossing regularly, until fragrant
- ➢ Add the mushrooms, carrot, sun-dried tomatoes (if using), and tomato paste
- ➢ Cook for 3 to 4 minutes over medium heat, tossing frequently, until fragrant
- ➢ Add the chickpeas, broth, wine, coriander (if using), and the sliced garlic
- ➢ Stir in the remaining ½ teaspoon ground turmeric
- ➢ Raise the heat, if needed, and bring to a boil, then lower heat to simmer
- ➢ Cover part of the way and let the sauce simmer for about 20 minutes, until thickened.
- ➢ Carefully add the seared fish to the skillet
- ➢ Ladle a bit of the sauce on top of the fish
- ➢ Add the artichokes, olives, lemon juice and slices, and rosemary sprigs
- ➢ Cook another 10 minutes or until the fish is fully cooked and flaky
- ➢ Garnish with fresh cilantro.

NUTRITION INFORMATION: Calories: 696 fat: 41g protein: 48g carbs: 37g fiber: 9g sodium: 810mg

114 INSTANT POT BLACK EYED PEAS

Servings: 4   **Cook Time: 25 Min**   **Prep Time 6 Min**

INGREDIENTS:

- ✓ 2 cups black-eyed peas (dried)
- ✓ 1 cup parsley, dill
- ✓ 2 slices oranges, 2 tbsp. tomato paste
- ✓ 4 green onions
- ✓ 2 carrots, bay leaves

DIRECTIONS:

- ➢ Clean the dill thoroughly with water removing stones.
- ➢ Add all the ingredients in the instant pot and stir well to combine.
- ➢ Lid the instant pot and set the vent to sealing.
- ➢ Set time for twenty-five minutes
- ➢ When the time has elapsed release pressure naturally.

NUTRITION INFORMATION: Calories: 506 Protein: 14g Carbohydrates: 33g

115 GREEN BEANS AND POTATOES IN OLIVE OIL

Servings: 4   **Cook Time: 17 Min**   **Prep Time 12 Min**

INGREDIENTS:

- ✓ 15 oz. tomatoes (diced)
- ✓ 2 potatoes
- ✓ 1 lb. green beans (fresh)
- ✓ 1 bunch dill, parsley, zucchini
- ✓ 1 tbsp. dried oregano

DIRECTIONS:

- ➢ Turn on the sauté function on your instant pot.
- ➢ Pour tomatoes, a cup of water and olive oil
- ➢ Add the rest of the ingredients and stir through.
- ➢ Lid the instant pot and set the valve to seal
- ➢ Set time for fifteen minutes.
- ➢ When the time has elapsed release pressure
- ➢ Remove the Fasolakia from the instant pot
- ➢ Serve and enjoy.

NUTRITION INFORMATION: Calories: 510 Protein: 20g Carbohydrates: 28g

116 BEEF STRIPS WITH LETTUCE SALAD

Servings: 5   **Cook Time: 12 Min**   **Prep Time 10 Min**

INGREDIENTS:

- ✓ 1 cup lettuce
- ✓ 10 oz. beef brisket
- ✓ 2 tablespoon sesame oil
- ✓ 1 tablespoon sunflower seeds
- ✓ 1 cucumber
- ✓ 1 teaspoon ground black pepper
- ✓ 1 teaspoon paprika
- ✓ 1 teaspoon Italian spices 2 teaspoon butter
- ✓ 1 teaspoon dried dill
- ✓ 2 tablespoon coconut milk

DIRECTIONS:

- ➢ Cut the beef brisket into strips.
- ➢ Sprinkle the beef strips with the ground black pepper, paprika, and dried dill.
- ➢ Preheat the air fryer to 365 F.
- ➢ Put the butter in the air fryer basket tray and melt it.
- ➢ Then add the beef strips and cook them for 6 minutes on each side.
- ➢ Meanwhile, tear the lettuce and toss it in a big salad bowl.
- ➢ Crush the sunflower seeds and sprinkle over the lettuce.
- ➢ Chop the cucumber into the small cubes and add to the salad bowl.
- ➢ Then combine the sesame oil and Italian spices together. Stir the oil.
- ➢ Combine the lettuce mixture with the coconut milk and stir it using 2 wooden spatulas.
- ➢ When the meat is cooked – let it chill to room temperature.
- ➢ Add the beef strips to the salad bowl.
- ➢ Stir it gently and sprinkle the salad with the sesame oil dressing.
- ➢ Serve the dish immediately.

NUTRITION INFORMATION: Calories: 199 Fat: 12.4g Carbs: 3.9g Protein: 18.1g

117 NUTRITIOUS VEGAN CABBAGE

Servings: 6 **Cook Time: 15 Min** **Prep Time 35 Min**

INGREDIENTS:

- ✓ 3 cups green cabbage
- ✓ 1 can tomatoes, onion
- ✓ Cups vegetable broth

- ✓ 3 stalks celery, carrots
- ✓ 2 tbsp. vinegar, sage

DIRECTIONS:

- ➢ Mix 1 tbsp. of lemon juice. 2 garlic cloves and the rest of ingredients in the instant pot and
- ➢ Lid and set time for fifteen minutes on high pressure.

- ➢ Release pressure naturally then remove the lid
- ➢ Remove the soup from the instant pot.
- ➢ Serve and enjoy.

NUTRITION INFORMATION: Calories: 67 Fat: 0.4g Fiber: 3.8g

118 INSTANT POT HORTA AND POTATOES

Servings: 4 **Cook Time: 17 Min** **Prep Time 12 Min**

INGREDIENTS:

- ✓ 2 heads of washed and chopped greens (spinach, Dandelion, kale, mustard green, Swiss chard)
- ✓ 6 potatoes (washed and cut in pieces)
- ✓ 1 cup virgin olive oil
- ✓ 1 lemon juice (reserve slices for serving)
- ✓ 10 garlic cloves (chopped)

DIRECTIONS:

- ➢ Position all the ingredients in the instant pot and lid setting the vent to sealing.
- ➢ Set time for fifteen minutes
- ➢ When time is done release pressure.
- ➢ Let the potatoes rest for some time
- ➢ Serve and enjoy with lemon slices.

NUTRITION INFORMATION: Calories: 499 Protein: 18g Carbohydrates: 41g

119 INSTANT POT JACKFRUIT CURRY

Servings: 2 **Cook Time: 16 Min** **Prep Time 1 H**

INGREDIENTS:

- ✓ 1 tbsp. oil
- ✓ Cumin seeds, Mustard seeds
- ✓ 2 tomatoes (purred)

- ✓ 20 oz. can green jackfruit (drained and rinsed)
- ✓ 1 tbsp. coriander powder, turmeric.

DIRECTIONS:

- ➢ Turn the instant pot to sauté mode
- ➢ Add cumin plus mustard seeds, then allow them to sizzle.
- ➢ Add other ingredients, and a cup of water then lid the instant pot

- ➢ Set time for seven minutes on high pressure.
- ➢ When the time has elapsed release pressure naturally
- ➢ Shred the jackfruit and serve.

NUTRITION INFORMATION: Calories: 369 Fat: 3g Fiber: 6g

120 BEAN FRITTATA WITH SWEET POTATOES

Servings: 4 **Cook Time: 20 Min** **Prep Time 25 Min**

INGREDIENTS:
- ✓ 4 eggs, whisked
- ✓ 1 red onion, chopped
- ✓ 2 tbsp olive oil
- ✓ 2 sweet potatoes, boiled and chopped
- ✓ ¾ cup ham, chopped
- ✓ ½ cup white beans, cooked
- ✓ 2 tbsp Greek yogurt Salt and black pepper to taste
- ✓ ½ cup cherry tomatoes, halved
- ✓ ¾ cup cheddar cheese, grated

DIRECTIONS:
- ➢ Warm the olive oil in a skillet over medium heat and sauté onion for 2 minutes
- ➢ Stir in sweet potatoes, ham, beans, yogurt, salt, pepper, and tomatoes
- ➢ Cook for another 3 minutes
- ➢ Pour in eggs and cheese, lock the lid
- ➢ Cook for an additional 10 minutes
- ➢ Cut before serving.

NUTRITION INFORMATION: Calories 280, Fat 18g, Carbs 9g, Protein 12g

121 SHRIMP WITH GARLIC AND MUSHROOMS

Servings: 4 **Cook Time: 15 Min** **Prep Time 10 Min**

INGREDIENTS:
- ✓ 1 pound (454 g) peeled and deveined fresh shrimp
- ✓ 1 teaspoon salt
- ✓ 1 cup extra-virgin olive oil
- ✓ 8 large garlic cloves, thinly sliced
- ✓ 4 ounces (113 g) sliced mushrooms (shiitake, baby bella, or button)
- ✓ ½ teaspoon red pepper flakes
- ✓ ¼ cup chopped fresh flat-leaf Italian parsley
- ✓ Zucchini noodles or riced cauliflower, for serving

DIRECTIONS:
- ➢ Rinse the shrimp and pat dry
- ➢ Place in a small bowl and sprinkle with the salt.
- ➢ In a large rimmed, thick skillet, heat the olive oil over medium-low heat
- ➢ Add the garlic and heat until very fragrant, 3 to 4 minutes
- ➢ Reduce the heat if the garlic starts to burn.
- ➢ Add the mushrooms and sauté for 5 minutes, until softened
- ➢ Then the shrimp and red pepper flakes and sauté
- ➢ (Until the shrimp begins to turn pink, another 3 to 4 minutes)
- ➢ Remove from the heat and stir in the parsley
- ➢ Serve over zucchini noodles or riced cauliflower.

NUTRITION INFORMATION: Calories: 620 fat: 56g protein: 24g carbs: 4g fiber: 0g sodium: 736mg

122 NACHOS

Servings: 4 **Cook Time: 10 Min** **Prep Time 5 Min**

INGREDIENTS:
- ✓ 4-ounce restaurant-style corn tortilla chips
- ✓ 1 medium green onion, thinly sliced (about 1 tbsp.)
- ✓ 1 (4 ounces) package finely crumbled feta cheese
- ✓ 1 finely chopped and drained plum tomato
- ✓ 2 tbsp Sun-dried tomatoes in oil, finely chopped
- ✓ 2 tbsp Kalamata olives

DIRECTIONS:
- ➢ Mix an onion, plum tomato, oil, sun-dried tomatoes, and olives in a small bowl.
- ➢ Arrange the tortillas chips on a microwavable plate in a single layer topped evenly with cheese
- ➢ (Microwave on high for one minute)
- ➢ Rotate the plate half turn and continue microwaving until the cheese is bubbly
- ➢ Spread the tomato mixture over the chips and cheese and enjoy.

NUTRITION INFORMATION: Calories: 140 Carbs: 19g Fat: 7g Protein: 2g

123 STUFFED CELERY

Servings: 3   **Cook Time: 20 Min**   **Prep Time 15 Min**

INGREDIENTS:

- ✓ Olive oil
- ✓ 1 clove garlic, minced 2 tbsp Pine nuts
- ✓ 2 tbsp dry-roasted sunflower seeds
- ✓ ¼ cup Italian cheese blend, shredded
- ✓ 8 stalks celery leaves
- ✓ 1 (8-ounce) fat-free cream cheese
- ✓ Cooking spray

DIRECTIONS:

- ➤ Sauté garlic and pine nuts over a medium setting for the heat
- ➤ (Until the nuts are golden brown)
- ➤ Cut off the wide base and tops from celery.
- ➤ Remove two thin strips from the round side of the celery to create a flat surface.
- ➤ Mix Italian cheese and cream cheese in a bowl
- ➤ Spread into cut celery stalks.
- ➤ Sprinkle half of the celery pieces with sunflower seeds and a half with the pine nut mixture
- ➤ Cover mixture and let stand for at least 4 hours before eating.

NUTRITION INFORMATION: Calories: 64 Carbs: 2g Fat: 6g Protein: 1g

124 CLASSIC ESCABECHE

Servings: 4   **Cook Time: 20 Min**   **Prep Time 10 Min**

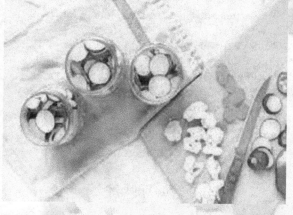

INGREDIENTS:

- ✓ 1 pound (454 g) wild-caught Spanish mackerel fillets, cut into four pieces
- ✓ 1 teaspoon salt
- ✓ ½ teaspoon freshly ground black pepper
- ✓ 8 tablespoons extra-virgin olive oil, divided
- ✓ 1 bunch asparagus, trimmed and cut into
- ✓ 2-inch pieces
- ✓ 1 (13¾-ounce / 390-g) can artichoke hearts, drained and quartered
- ✓ 4 large garlic cloves, peeled and crushed
- ✓ 2 bay leaves
- ✓ ¼ cup red wine vinegar
- ✓ ½ teaspoon smoked paprika

DIRECTIONS:

- ➤ Sprinkle the fillets with salt and pepper and let sit at room temperature for 5 minutes.
- ➤ In a large skillet, heat 2 tablespoons olive oil over medium-high heat
- ➤ Add the fish, skin-side up, and cook 5 minutes
- ➤ Flip and cook 5 minutes on the other side, until browned and cooked through
- ➤ Transfer to a serving dish, pour the cooking oil over the fish, and cover to keep warm.
- ➤ Heat the remaining 6 tablespoons olive oil in the same skillet over medium heat
- ➤ Add the asparagus, artichokes, garlic, and bay
- ➤ Leaves and sauté until the vegetables are tender, 6 to 8 minutes.
- ➤ Use slotted spoon
- ➤ Top the fish with the cooked vegetables, reserving the oil in the skillet
- ➤ Then the vinegar and paprika to the oil and whisk to combine well
- ➤ Pour the vinaigrette over the fish and vegetables
- ➤ Let sit at room temperature for at least 15 minutes
- ➤ (Or marinate in the refrigerator up to 24 hours for a deeper flavor)
- ➤ Remove the bay leaf before serving.

NUTRITION INFORMATION: Calories: 578 fat: 50g protein: 26g carbs: 13g fiber: 5g sodium: 946mg

125 OLIVE OIL-POACHED TUNA

Servings: 4   **Cook Time: 45 Min**   **Prep Time 15 Min**

INGREDIENTS:

- ✓ 1 cup extra-virgin olive oil, plus more if needed
- ✓ 4 (3- to 4-inch) sprigs fresh rosemary
- ✓ 8 (3- to 4-inch) sprigs fresh thyme
- ✓ 2 large garlic cloves, thinly sliced
- ✓ 2 (2-inch) strips lemon zest
- ✓ 1 teaspoon salt
- ✓ ½ teaspoon freshly ground black pepper
- ✓ 1 pound (454 g) fresh tuna steaks (about 1 inch thick)

DIRECTIONS:

- ➤ Select a thick pot just large enough to fit the tuna in a single layer on the bottom
- ➤ The larger the pot, the more olive oil you will need to use
- ➤ Combine the olive oil, rosemary, thyme, garlic, lemon zest, salt, and pepper over medium-low heat
- ➤ Cook until warm and fragrant, 20 to 25 minutes, lowering the heat if it begins to smoke.
- ➤ Remove from the heat and allow to cool for 25 to 30 minutes, until warm but not hot.
- ➤ Add the tuna to the bottom of the pan, adding additional oil if needed
- ➤ So that tuna is fully submerged, and return to medium-low heat
- ➤ Cook for 5 to 10 minutes
- ➤ (Or until the oil heats back up and is warm and fragrant but not smoking)
- ➤ Lower the heat if it gets too hot.
- ➤ Remove the pot from the heat and let the tuna cook in warm oil 4 to 5 minutes, to your desired level of doneness
- ➤ For a tuna that is rare in the center, cook for 2 to 3 minutes.
- ➤ Remove from the oil and serve warm, drizzling 2 to 3 tablespoons seasoned oil over the tuna.
- ➤ To store for later use, remove the tuna from the oil
- ➤ Place in a container with a lid
- ➤ Allow tuna and oil to cool separately. When both have cooled
- ➤ Remove the herb stems with a slotted spoon and pour the cooking oil over the tuna
- ➤ Cover and store in the refrigerator for up to 1 week
- ➤ Bring to room temperature to allow the oil to liquify before serving.

NUTRITION INFORMATION: Calories: 363 fat: 28g protein: 27g carbs: 1g fiber: 0g sodium: 624mg

126 ITALIAN SPINACH & RICE SALAD

Servings: 2   **Cook Time: 45 Min**   **Prep Time 30 Min**

INGREDIENTS:

- ✓ 1 tbsp olive oil Salt and black pepper to taste
- ✓ ½ cup baby spinach ½ cup green peas, blanched
- ✓ 1 garlic clove, minced ½ cup white rice, rinsed
- ✓ ½ cup cherry tomatoes, halved
- ✓ 1 tbsp parsley, chopped
- ✓ 2 tbsp Italian salad dressing

DIRECTIONS:

- ➤ Bring a large pot of salted water to a boil over medium heat
- ➤ Pour in the rice, cover, and simmer on a low heat for 15-18 minutes
- ➤ (Or until until the rice is al dente)
- ➤ Drain and let cool into a salad bowl
- ➤ In a bowl, whisk the olive oil, garlic, salt, and black pepper
- ➤ Toss the green peas, baby spinach, and rice together
- ➤ Pour the dressing all over and gently stir to combine
- ➤ Decorate with cherry tomatoes and parsley and serve. Enjoy!

NUTRITION INFORMATION: Calories 160, Fat 14g, Carbs 9g, Protein 4g

127 FRUITY ASPARAGUS-QUINOA SALAD

Servings: 8 **Cook Time: 25 Min** **Prep Time 25 Min**

INGREDIENTS:

- ¼ cup chopped pecans, toasted
- ½ cup finely chopped white onion
- ½ jalapeno pepper, diced
- ½ lb. asparagus, sliced to
- 2-inch lengths, steamed and chilled
- ½ tsp kosher salt
- 1 cup fresh orange sections
- 1 cup uncooked quinoa
- 1 tsp olive oil
- 2 cups water
- 2 tbsp minced red onion
- 5 dates, pitted and chopped

- 2 tbsp chopped fresh mint
- 2 tbsp fresh lemon juice Mint sprigs(optional)

DRESSING INGREDIENTS:

- ¼ tsp ground black pepper
- ¼ tsp kosher salt 1 garlic clove, minced
- 1 tbsp olive oil

DIRECTIONS:

- Wash and rub with your hands the quinoa in a bowl at least three times, discarding water each and every time
- On medium high fire, place a large nonstick fry pan and heat 1 tsp olive oil
- For two minutes, sauté onions before adding quinoa and sautéing for another five minutes
- Add ½ tsp salt and 2 cups water and bring to a boil

- Lower fire to a simmer, cover and cook for 15 minutes
- Turn off fire and let stand until water is absorbed
- Then pepper asparagus, dates, pecans and orange sections into a salad bowl
- Join also cooked quinoa, toss to mix well
- In a small bowl, whisk mint, garlic, black pepper, salt, olive oil and lemon juice to create the dressing
- Pour dressing over salad, serve and enjoy.

NUTRITION INFORMATION: Calories: 173; Fat: 6.3g; Protein: 4.3g; Carbohydrates: 24.7g

128 ZA'ATAR SALMON WITH CUCUMBER SALAD

Servings: 4 **Cook Time: 25 Min** **Prep Time 5 Min**

INGREDIENTS:

SALAD
- 4 cups sliced cucumber
- 1 pint cherry tomatoes, halved
- 1/4 cup chopped fresh dill

SALMON:
- 11/2 pounds (680 g) skinless salmon
- 1 tablespoon Za'atar

- 1/4 cup cider vinegar
- 1/4 teaspoon salt
- 1/4 teaspoon black pepper

- 4 lemon wedges

DIRECTIONS:

- Preheat the oven to 350°F (180°C). Line a baking sheet with aluminum foil.
- Toss all the salad ingredients in a bowl until combined. Set aside.
- Season the salmon with Za'atar on both sides

- Place on the prepared baking sheet. Roast in the preheated oven for about 25 minutes
- (Or until the internal temperature registers 145°F (63°C))
- Serve the salmon with the salad and lemon wedges.

NUTRITION INFORMATION: 1 Lean 3 Greens 3 Condiments

129 GARDEN SALAD WITH ORANGES AND OLIVES

Servings: 4　　　　　**Cook Time: 15 Min**　　　　　**Prep Time 15 Min**

INGREDIENTS:

- ½ cup red wine vinegar
- 1 tbsp extra virgin olive oil
- 1 tbsp finely chopped celery
- 1 tbsp finely chopped red onion
- 16 large ripe black olives
- 2 garlic cloves

- 2 navel oranges, peeled and segmented
- 4 boneless, skinless chicken breasts
- 4-oz each 4 garlic cloves, minced
- 8 cups leaf lettuce, washed and dried
- Cracked black pepper to taste

DIRECTIONS:

- Prepare the dressing by mixing pepper, celery, onion, olive oil, garlic and vinegar in a small bowl
- Whisk well to combine. Lightly grease grate and preheat grill to high
- Rub chicken with the garlic cloves and discard garlic
- Grill chicken for 5 minutes per side or until cooked through

- Remove from grill and let it stand for 5 minutes before cutting into ½-inch strips
- In 4 serving plates, evenly arrange two cups lettuce, ¼ of the sliced oranges and 4 olives per plate
- Top each plate with ¼ serving of grilled chicken, evenly drizzle with dressing
- Serve and enjoy.

NUTRITION INFORMATION: Calories: 259.8; Protein: 48.9g; Carbs: 12.9g; Fat: 1.4g

130 CAULIFLOWER GRITS, SHRIMP AND CREAMY

Servings: 2　　　　　**Cook Time: 15 Min**　　　　　**Prep Time 10 Min**

INGREDIENTS:

- 1 pound (454 g) raw, peeled and deveined shrimp
- 1/2 tablespoon Cajun seasoning
- Cooking spray
- 1/4 cup chicken broth
- 1 tablespoon lemon juice
- 1 tablespoon butter

- 2 1/2 cups finely riced cauliflower
- 1/2 cup unsweetened almond or cashew milk
- 1/4 teaspoon salt
- 1/3 cup reduced-fat shredded Cheddar cheese
- 2 tablespoons sour cream
- 1/4 cup thinly sliced scallions

DIRECTIONS:

- Add the shrimp and Cajun seasoning into a large, resealable plastic bag
- Seal the bag and toss to coat well.
- Grease a skillet with cooking spray and heat over medium heat.
- Then the shrimp and cook each side for about 2 to 3 minutes
- Join also chicken broth and lemon juice, scraping any bits off of the bottom of the pan
- Let simmer for 1 minute. Remove from the heat and set aside

- In a separate skillet, melt the butter over medium heat.
- Add the riced cauliflower and cook for 5 minutes
- Then milk and salt and cook for an additional 5 minutes.
- Remove from heat and stir in sour cream and cheese until melted.
- Serve the shrimp over cauliflower grits and sprinkle with the scallions.

NUTRITION INFORMATION: 1 Leanest 3 Greens 2 Healthy Fats 3 Condiments

131 CHICKEN WITH SWIMMING RAMA

Servings: 4 **Cook Time: 10 Min** **Prep Time 10 Min**

INGREDIENTS:

- ✓ 2 pounds chicken breast tenders or chicken breasts cut into
- ✓ 1-2 inch strips
- ✓ 8 wooden or metal kebab skewers
- ✓ 2 teaspoons turmeric
- ✓ 1 cup Coconut Milk, divided
- ✓ 1/4 cup powdered peanut butter
- ✓ 1 tablespoon soy sauce
- ✓ 1 teaspoon grated fresh ginger
- ✓ 1 packet stevia or other non-calorie sweetener
- ✓ 2 1/2 cups of your favorite low-carbohydrate stir-fry vegetables cut into bite size pieces
- ✓ (Use broccoli, cabbage, radishes, mushrooms, and peppers)

DIRECTIONS:

- ➤ Combine 1/4 cup of coconut milk and turmeric and pour over chicken
- ➤ Allow to marinate 4 hours or overnight.
- ➤ If using wooden skewers, allow to soak in water while chicken is marinating.
- ➤ Pat dry chicken. Divide chicken between skewers and set aside
- ➤ In a saucepan over medium heat combine remaining coconut milk, Peanut Butter, soy sauce and sweetener
- ➤ Stir until warmed through.
- ➤ Heat grill to high heat and grill chicken skewers 3 minutes on each side.
- ➤ Meanwhile, steam or water-sauté vegetables.
- ➤ Divide vegetables among four plates
- ➤ Top each with 2 chicken skewers and pour peanut sauce over the top.

NUTRITION INFORMATION: 325 calories, 7 grams of carbohydrates, 7 grams of fat, and 55

132 DAIKON NOODLE SALAD

Servings: 4 **Cook Time: 0 Min** **Prep Time 10 Min**

INGREDIENTS:

- ✓ 4 cups daikon radish, julienned or spiralized (see Basics: Specialized Tools)
- ✓ 1 teaspoon hot chili sauce
- ✓ 2 tablespoons lime

DIRECTIONS:

- ➤ Toss all ingredients together and chill

NUTRITION INFORMATION: 331 calories, 7 grams of carbohydrates, 4 grams of fat, and 66 grams of protein.

133 MASALA CHICKEN

Servings: 4   **Cook Time: 40 Min**   **Prep Time 10 Min**

INGREDIENTS:

- ✓ 1 1/2 pounds boneless skinless chicken breast, cut in large chunks
- ✓ 2 tablespoons butter
- ✓ 2 teaspoons masala
- ✓ 1 tablespoon grated fresh ginger
- ✓ 2 cups canned diced tomatoes, undrained
- ✓ 1 cup chopped leeks
- ✓ 1 cup yellow squash chopped
- ✓ 2 cups cauliflower florets Salt to taste
- ✓ 1 cup plain Greek yogurt
- ✓ 1 cup chopped cilantro

DIRECTIONS:

- ➢ Spray a nonstick pan with cooking spray and heat over medium high heat.
- ➢ Add chicken and brown on all sides.
- ➢ Remove from pan and set aside.
- ➢ Reduce heat and add the butter, spices, and vegetables
- ➢ Cook, stirring occasionally
- ➢ (Until vegetables are tender and tomatoes are reduced, approximately 40 minutes)
- ➢ Remove about 1 cup of the vegetables from the pan
- ➢ Blend until smooth. Salt to taste
- ➢ Return blended vegetables and chicken to pan
- ➢ Heat until chicken is warmed through, approximately 10 minutes.
- ➢ Remove from heat and stir in 1/2 cup yogurt.
- ➢ Top with additional yogurt and cilantro.

NUTRITION INFORMATION: 311 calories, 11 grams of carbohydrates, 8 grams of fat, and 47 grams of protein.

134 FIVE-SPICE MEATBALLS

Servings: 4   **Cook Time: 30 Min**   **Prep Time 10 Min**

INGREDIENTS:

- ✓ 2 packages 99% lean ground turkey (20 oz. each)
- ✓ 1 cup ground meat mix (see Basics: Ground Meat Mix)
- ✓ 1 teaspoon ground five-spice
- ✓ 4 teaspoons Olive oil 1 clove minced garlic
- ✓ 1/2 teaspoon salt
- ✓ 4 cups baby bok choy, or bok choy cut into
- ✓ 1-inch pieces

DIRECTIONS:

- ➢ Preheat oven to 425°. Cover a baking sheet with foil.
- ➢ Combine ground turkey, ground meat mix, five-spice and salt
- ➢ Roll into one inch balls
- ➢ Place on foil-lined baking sheet.
- ➢ Bake 30 minutes or until cooked through.
- ➢ Remove pan from oven and set aside.
- ➢ Heat heavy-bottomed pan or wok to high
- ➢ Add 2 tablespoons of peanut oil and swirl around bottom of pan
- ➢ Then garlic and bok choy and stir fry quickly
- ➢ (Until bok choy is browned and heated through)
- ➢ Divide among 4 plates and top with meatballs.

NUTRITION INFORMATION: 354 Calories, 3 grams of carbohydrates, 9 grams of fat, and 67 grams of protein.

135 CHICKEN DIVAN

Servings: 4   **Cook Time: 25 Min**   **Prep Time 10 Min**

INGREDIENTS:

- 18 oz. cooked turkey or chicken breast, chopped into
- 1-inch cubes
- 1 1/2 cups low-fat blend (see Basics: Low-Fat Blend)
- 1/2 tsp. chicken-flavored Better Than Bouillon
- 1/4 cup minced onion

- 2 teaspoons Dijon mustard
- 1 teaspoon dried thyme
- 1/4 cup light mayo
- 1 cup frozen broccoli florets
- 1 cup mushrooms, sliced
- 4 cups yellow summer squash
- 1/4 cup Parmesan cheese

DIRECTIONS:

- Preheat oven to 375°
- Spray large casserole with nonstick cooking spray.
- Use a vegetable peeler, peel squash into long thin strips as wide as you can
- Discard center seeds. Roll in several layers of paper towels
- Squeeze out as much of the water as possible. Set aside.

- Blend low-fat blend, mayo, bouillon concentrate, minced onion, mustard, and thyme
- Fold in chicken and vegetables.
- Pour into prepared baking dish
- Sprinkle with Parmesan
- Bake 25 minutes or until warmed through.
- Let cool 10 minutes before serving.

NUTRITION INFORMATION: 299 calories, 12 grams of carbohydrates, 8 grams of fat, and 47 grams of protein.

136 BUTTERNUT SQUASH FRIES

Servings: 2   **Cook Time: 10 Min**   **Prep Time 5 Min**

INGREDIENTS:

- 1 Butternut squash
- 1 tbsp Extra virgin olive oil
- ½ tbsp Grapeseed oil
- 1/8 tsp Sea salt

DIRECTIONS:

- Remove seeds from the squash and cut into thin slices
- Coat with extra virgin olive oil and grapeseed oil
- Add a sprinkle of salt and toss to coat well.
- Arrange the squash slices onto three baking sheets
- Bake for 10 minutes until crispy.

NUTRITION INFORMATION: Calories: 40 Carbs: 10g Fat: 0g Protein: 1g

137 DRIED FIG TAPENADE

Serving: 1   **Cook Time: 0 Min**   **Prep Time 5 Min**

INGREDIENTS:

- 1 cup Dried figs
- 1 cup Kalamata olives
- ½ cup Water

- 1 tbsp Chopped fresh thyme
- 1 tbsp extra virgin olive oil
- ½ tsp Balsamic vinegar

DIRECTIONS:

- Prepare figs in a food processor until well chopped
- Add water, and continue processing to form a paste.
- Then olives and pulse until well blended

- Join also. Add thyme, vinegar, and extra virgin olive oil
- Pulse until very smooth. Best served with crackers of your choice

NUTRITION INFORMATION: Calories: 249 Carbs: 64g Fat: 1g Protein: 3g

138 FIDEOS WITH SEAFOOD

Servings: 8 **Cook Time: 20 Min** **Prep Time 15 Min**

INGREDIENTS:
- ✓ 1 tablespoons extra-virgin olive oil, plus
- ✓ ½ cup, divided
- ✓ 6 cups zucchini noodles, roughly chopped (2 to 3 medium zucchini)
- ✓ 1 pound (454 g) shrimp, peeled, deveined and roughly chopped
- ✓ 6 to 8 ounces (170 to 227 g) canned chopped clams, drained
- ✓ 4 ounces (113 g) crab meat
- ✓ ½ cup crumbled goat cheese
- ✓ ½ cup crumbled feta cheese
- ✓ 1 (28-ounce / 794-g) can chopped tomatoes, with their juices
- ✓ 1 teaspoon salt
- ✓ 1 teaspoon garlic powder
- ✓ ½ teaspoon smoked paprika
- ✓ ½ cup shredded Parmesan cheese
- ✓ ¼ cup chopped fresh flat-leaf Italian parsley, for garnish

DIRECTIONS:
- ➢ Preheat the oven to 375°F (190°C).
- ➢ Pour 2 tablespoons olive oil in the bottom of a 9-by-13-inch baking dish and swirl to coat the bottom.
- ➢ In a large bowl, combine the zucchini noodles, shrimp, clams, and crab meat.
- ➢ In another bowl, combine the goat cheese, feta, and ¼ cup olive oil and stir to combine well
- ➢ Add the canned tomatoes and their juices, salt, garlic powder, and paprika and combine well.
- ➢ Then the mixture to the zucchini and seafood mixture and stir to combine.
- ➢ Pour the mixture into the prepared baking dish, spreading evenly
- ➢ Spread shredded Parmesan over top
- ➢ Drizzle with the remaining ¼ cup olive oil
- ➢ Bake until bubbly, 20 to 25 minutes
- ➢ Serve warm, garnished with chopped parsley.

NUTRITION INFORMATION: Calories: 434 fat: 31g protein: 29g carbs: 12g fiber: 3g sodium: 712mg

139 SHRIMP PESTO RICE BOWLS

Servings: 4 **Cook Time: 5 Min** **Prep Time 5 Min**

INGREDIENTS:
- ✓ 1 pound (454 g) medium shrimp, peeled and deveined
- ✓ ¼ cup pesto sauce
- ✓ 1 lemon, sliced
- ✓ 2 cups cooked wild rice pilaf

DIRECTIONS:
- ➢ Preheat the air fryer to 360°F (182°C).
- ➢ In a medium bowl, toss the shrimp with the pesto sauce until well coated.
- ➢ Place the shrimp in a single layer in the air fryer basket
- ➢ Put the lemon slices over the shrimp and roast for 5 minutes.
- ➢ Remove the lemons and discard
- ➢ Serve a quarter of the shrimp over ½ cup wild rice with some favorite steamed vegetables.

NUTRITION INFORMATION: Calories: 249 fat: 10g protein: 20g carbs: 20g fiber: 2g sodium: 277mg

140 SALMON WITH TOMATOES AND OLIVES

Servings: 4   Cook Time: 8 Min   Prep Time 5 Min

INGREDIENTS:

- ✓ 2 tablespoons olive oil
- ✓ 4 (1½-inch-thick) salmon fillets
- ✓ ½ teaspoon salt
- ✓ ¼ teaspoon cayenne
- ✓ 1 teaspoon chopped fresh dill
- ✓ 2 Roma tomatoes, diced
- ✓ ¼ cup sliced Kalamata olives 4 lemon slices

DIRECTIONS:

- ➤ Preheat the air fryer to 380°F (193°C).
- ➤ Brush the olive oil on both sides of the salmon fillets
- ➤ Then season them lightly with salt, cayenne, and dill.
- ➤ Place the fillets in a single layer in the basket of the air fryer
- ➤ Layer the tomatoes and olives over the top
- ➤ Top each fillet with a lemon slice.
- ➤ Bake for 8 minutes
- ➤ (Or until the salmon has reached an internal temperature of 145°F (63°C)).

NUTRITION INFORMATION: Calories: 241 fat: 15g protein: 23g carbs: 3g fiber: 1g sodium: 595mg

141 BAKED TROUT WITH LEMON

Servings: 4   Cook Time: 15 Min   Prep Time 5 Min

INGREDIENTS:

- ✓ 4 trout fillets
- ✓ 2 tablespoons olive oil
- ✓ ½ teaspoon salt
- ✓ 1 teaspoon black pepper
- ✓ 2 garlic cloves, sliced
- ✓ 1 lemon, sliced, plus additional wedges for serving

DIRECTIONS:

- ➤ Preheat the air fryer to 380°F (193°C).
- ➤ Brush each fillet with olive oil on both sides
- ➤ Season with salt and pepper
- ➤ Place the fillets in an even layer in the air fryer basket.
- ➤ Place the sliced garlic over the tops of the trout fillets
- ➤ then top the garlic with lemon slices
- ➤ Cook for 12 to 15 minutes
- ➤ (Or until it has reached an internal temperature of 145°F (63°C))
- ➤ Serve with fresh lemon wedges.

NUTRITION INFORMATION: Calories: 231 fat: 12g protein: 29g carbs: 1g fiber: 0g sodium: 341mg

142 SPEEDY SWEET POTATO CHIPS

Servings: 4   Cook Time: 0 Min   Prep Time 15 Min

INGREDIENTS:

- ✓ 1 large Sweet potato
- ✓ 1 tbsp Extra virgin olive oil
- ✓ Salt

DIRECTIONS:

- ➤ 300°F preheated oven. Slice your potato into nice, thin slices that resemble fries.
- ➤ Toss the potato slices with salt and extra virgin olive oil in a bowl
- ➤ Bake for about one hour, flipping every 15 minutes until crispy and browned

NUTRITION INFORMATION: Calories: 150 Carbs: 16g Fat: 9g Protein: 1g

143 NACHOS WITH HUMMUS (MEDITERRANEAN INSPIRED)

Servings: 4   **Cook Time: 20 Min**   **Prep Time 15 Min**

INGREDIENTS:

- ✓ 4 cups salted pita chips
- ✓ 1 (8 oz.) red pepper (roasted) Hummus
- ✓ 1 tsp Finely shredded lemon peel
- ✓ ¼ cup Chopped pitted Kalamata olives
- ✓
- ✓ ¼ cup crumbled feta cheese
- ✓ 1 plum (Roma) tomato, seeded, chopped
- ✓ ½ cup chopped cucumber
- ✓ 1 tsp Chopped fresh oregano leaves

DIRECTIONS:

- ➤ 400°F preheated oven
- ➤ Arrange the pita chips on a heatproof platter and drizzle with hummus.
- ➤ Top with olives, tomato, cucumber, cheese
- ➤ Bake until warmed through
- ➤ Sprinkle lemon zest and oregano and enjoy while it's hot.

NUTRITION INFORMATION: Calories: 130 Carbs: 18g Fat: 5g Protein: 4g

144 SEA SCALLOPS WITH WHITE BEAN PURÉE

Servings: 2   **Cook Time: 10 Min**   **Prep Time 10 Min**

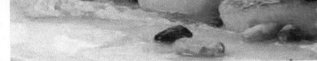

INGREDIENTS:

- ✓ 4 tablespoons olive oil, divided 2 garlic cloves
- ✓ 2 teaspoons minced fresh rosemary
- ✓ 1 (15-ounce / 425-g) can white cannellini beans, drained and rinsed
- ✓ ½ cup low-sodium chicken stock
- ✓ Salt, to taste
- ✓ Freshly ground black pepper, to taste
- ✓ 6 (10 ounce / 283-g) sea scallops

DIRECTIONS:

- ➤ To make the bean purée, heat 2 tablespoons of olive oil in a saucepan over medium-high heat
- ➤ Add the garlic and sauté for 30 seconds, or just until it's fragrant
- ➤ Don't let it burn
- ➤ Then the rosemary and remove the pan from the heat.
- ➤ Add the white beans and chicken stock to the pan, return it to the heat, and stir
- ➤ Bring the beans to a boil
- ➤ Reduce the heat to low and simmer for 5 minutes.
- ➤ Transfer the beans to a blender and purée them for 30 seconds, or until they're smooth
- ➤ Taste and season with salt and pepper
- ➤ Let them sit in the blender with the lid on to keep them warm while you prepare the scallops.
- ➤ Pat the scallops dry with a paper towel
- ➤ Season them with salt and pepper.
- ➤ Heat the remaining 2 tablespoons of olive oil in a large sauté pan
- ➤ When the oil is shimmering, add the scallops, flat-side down.
- ➤ Cook the scallops for 2 minutes, or until they're golden on the bottom
- ➤ Flip them over and cook for another 1 to 2 minutes, or until opaque and slightly firm.
- ➤ To serve, divide the bean purée between two plates and top with the scallops.

NUTRITION INFORMATION: Calories: 465 fat: 28g protein: 30g carbs: 21g fiber: 7g sodium: 319mg

145 GREEN CHILI ENCHILADAS

Servings: 4 **Cook Time: 30 Min** **Prep Time 10 Min**

INGREDIENTS:

- ✓ 14 oz. canned roasted green chilies (not jalapenos), divided
- ✓ 13 oz. canned tomatillos, drain and rinsed
- ✓ 1/2 cup leeks, chopped
- ✓ 1 cup cilantro, finely chopped, divided

- ✓ 2 cloves garlic, minced
- ✓ 12 oz. shredded low-fat cheese
- ✓ 3/4 cup 2% cottage cheese, blended until smooth
- ✓ 1/2 cup chopped mild onion
- ✓ 8 oz. turkey breast cutlets

DIRECTIONS:

- ➤ Preheat oven to 400°. Spray 9x11 baking dish with nonstick cooking spray.
- ➤ Place turkey breast cutlets between two pieces of plastic wrap
- ➤ Use a meat mallet or rolling pin, pound turkey cutlet until very thin. Set aside.
- ➤ For sauce, blend green chilies, tomatillos, leeks, 1/2 cup of cilantro, and garlic gloves until smooth. Set aside.

- ➤ For filling, combine remaining chilies, 8 oz. of shredded cheese, cottage cheese, and onion.
- ➤ Use turkey cutlet like a tortilla shell, divide filling among cutlets, roll up cutlets to form rolls
- ➤ Place seam-side down in baking dish.
- ➤ Pour sauce over cutlets, top with remaining cheese and bake 30 minutes uncovered.
- ➤ Top with remaining cilantro and serve.

NUTRITION INFORMATION: 278 Calories, 14 grams of carbohydrates, 12 grams of fat, and 25 grams of protein.

146 VEGETABLE TORTILLAS

Servings: 4 **Cook Time: 7 Min** **Prep Time 15 Min**

INGREDIENTS:

- ✓ 2 zucchinis, cut in half, then sliced
- ✓ 1/2 inch thick 1 leek, washed and sliced
- ✓ 1 bunch scallions, cut into
- ✓ 1/2-inch pieces
- ✓ 1/4 pound (113 g) mushrooms, sliced
- ✓ 1 cup small broccoli florets
- ✓ ¾ cup water, divided
- ✓ 1 (7-0unce / 198-g) can Mexican green sauce
- ✓ 1/8 cup packed chopped fresh cilantro
- ✓ 1 tablespoon cornstarch, mixed with
- ✓ 2 tablespoons water
- ✓ 8 whole-wheat flour tortillas

DIRECTIONS:

- ➤ In a pan over medium heat, sauté the zucchinis, leek, scallions, mushrooms
- ➤ Then broccoli florets in 1/2 cup of the water for 5 minutes, or until tender-crisp.
- ➤ Stir in the remaining 1/4 cup of the water, green sauce and cilantro

- ➤ Pour in the cornstarch mixture
- ➤ Cook for 2 minutes, stirring constantly, or until thickened.
- ➤ Place a line of the vegetable mixture down the center of a tortilla
- ➤ Roll up and serve.

NUTRITION INFORMATION: Calories: 410 fat: 9.1g carbs: 73.1g protein: 11.2g fiber: 11.3g

147 SWEET POTATO AND MUSHROOM SKILLET

Servings: 4   **Cook Time: 15 Min**   **Prep Time 5 Min**

INGREDIENTS:
- ✓ 1 cup low-sodium vegetable broth
- ✓ 8 ounces (227 g) mushrooms, sliced
- ✓ 4 medium sweet potatoes, cut into
- ✓ 1/2-inch dice 1 sweet onion, diced
- ✓ 1 bell pepper, diced
- ✓ 1 teaspoon garlic powder
- ✓ 1/2 teaspoon chili powder
- ✓ 1/2 teaspoon ground cumin
- ✓ 1/8 teaspoon freshly ground black pepper

DIRECTIONS:
- ➢ Heat a large skillet over medium-low heat
- ➢ Stir in all the ingredients
- ➢ Cover and cook for 10 minutes
- ➢ (Or until the sweet potatoes are easily pierced with a fork)
- ➢ Uncover and give the mixture a good stir
- ➢ Cook, uncovered, for an additional 5 minutes, stirring once halfway through.
- ➢ Serve hot.

NUTRITION INFORMATION: Calories: 159 fat: 1.2g carbs: 33.9g protein: 6.2g fiber: 5.9g

148 SAUTÉED COLLARD GREENS

Servings: 4   **Cook Time: 25 Min**   **Prep Time 10 Min**

INGREDIENTS:
- ✓ 11/2 pounds (680 g) collard greens
- ✓ 1 cup low-sodium vegetable broth
- ✓ 1/2 teaspoon onion powder
- ✓ 1/2 teaspoon garlic powder
- ✓ 1/8 teaspoon freshly ground black pepper

DIRECTIONS:
- ➢ Remove the hard middle stems from the greens and roughly
- ➢ Chop the leaves into 2-inch pieces.
- ➢ In a large saucepan over medium-high heat
- ➢ Combine all the ingredients, except for the collard greens.
- ➢ Bring to a boil, then add the chopped greens
- ➢ Reduce the heat to low and cover.
- ➢ Cook for 20 minutes, stirring constantly.
- ➢ Serve warm.

NUTRITION INFORMATION: Calories: 528 fat: 55.1g carbs: 8.8g protein: 3.2g fiber: 2.3g

149 HUMMUS AND OLIVE PITA BREAD

Servings: 3   **Cook Time: 0 Min**   **Prep Time 5 Min**

INGREDIENTS:
- ✓ 7 pita bread cut into 6 wedges each
- ✓ 1 (7 ounces) container plain hummus
- ✓ 1 tbsp Greek vinaigrette
- ✓ ½ cup Chopped pitted Kalamata olives

DIRECTIONS:
- ➢ Spread the hummus on a serving plate
- ➢ Mix vinaigrette and olives in a bowl and spoon over the hummus
- ➢ Enjoy with wedges of pita bread.

NUTRITION INFORMATION: Calories: 225 Carbs: 40g Fat: 5g Protein: 9g

150 ROAST ASPARAGUS

Servings: 4 **Cook Time: 5 Min** **Prep Time 15 Min**

INGREDIENTS:

- ✓ 1 tbsp Extra virgin olive oil (1 tablespoon)
- ✓ 1 medium lemon
- ✓ ½ tsp Freshly grated nutmeg
- ✓ ½ tsp black pepper
- ✓ ½ tsp Kosher salt

DIRECTIONS:

- ➢ Warm the oven to 500°F
- ➢ Put the asparagus on an aluminum foil
- ➢ Drizzle with extra virgin olive oil, and toss until well coated.
- ➢ Roast the asparagus in the oven for about five minutes
- ➢ Toss and continue roasting until browned
- ➢ Sprinkle the roasted asparagus with nutmeg, salt, zest, and pepper.

NUTRITION INFORMATION: Calories: 123 Carbs: 5g Fat: 11g Protein: 3g

151 FISH FILLET ON LEMONS

Servings: 4 **Cook Time: 6 Min** **Prep Time 5 Min**

INGREDIENTS:

- ✓ 4 (4-ounce/ 113-g) fish fillets, such as tilapia, salmon, catfish, cod, or your favorite fish
- ✓ Nonstick cooking spray
- ✓ 3 to 4 medium lemons
- ✓ 1 tablespoon extra-virgin olive oil
- ✓ ¼ teaspoon freshly ground black pepper
- ✓ ¼ teaspoon kosher or sea salt

DIRECTIONS:

- ➢ Use paper towels, pat the fillets dry and let stand at room temperature for 10 minutes
- ➢ Meanwhile, coat the cold cooking grate of the grill with nonstick cooking spray
- ➢ Preheat the grill to 400°F (205°C), or medium-high heat
- ➢ Or preheat a grill pan over medium-high heat on the stove top.
- ➢ Cut one lemon in half and set half aside
- ➢ Slice the remaining half of that lemon and the remaining lemons into ¼-inch-thick slices
- ➢ (You should have about 12 to 16 lemon slices.)
- ➢ Into a small bowl, squeeze 1 tablespoon of juice out of the reserved lemon half.
- ➢ Add the oil to the bowl with the lemon juice
- ➢ Mix well. Brush both sides of the fish with the oil mixture
- ➢ Sprinkle evenly with pepper and salt.
- ➢ Carefully place the lemon slices on the grill (or the grill pan)
- ➢ Arrange 3 to 4 slices together in the shape of a fish fillet
- ➢ Repeat with the remaining slices
- ➢ Place the fish fillets directly on top of the lemon slices
- ➢ Grill with the lid closed
- ➢ (If you're grilling on the stove top, cover with a large pot lid or aluminum foil.)
- ➢ Turn the fish halfway through the cooking time
- ➢ (Only if the fillets are more than half an inch thick)
- ➢ The fish is done and ready to serve
- ➢ (When it just begins to separate into flakes (chunks) when pressed gently with a fork).

NUTRITION INFORMATION: Calories: 208 fat: 11g protein: 21g carbs: 2g fiber: 0g sodium: 249mg

152 PANKO-CRUSTED FISH STICKS

Servings: 4   **Cook Time: 5 Min**   **Prep Time 10 Min**

INGREDIENTS:

- ✓ 2 large eggs, lightly beaten
- ✓ 1 tablespoon 2% milk
- ✓ 1 pound (454 g) skinned fish fillets (cod, tilapia, or other white fish) about ½ inch thick, sliced into 20 (1-inch-wide) strips
- ✓ ½ cup yellow cornmeal
- ✓ ½ cup whole-wheat panko bread crumbs or whole-wheat bread crumbs
- ✓ ¼ teaspoon smoked paprika
- ✓ ¼ teaspoon kosher or sea salt
- ✓ ¼ teaspoon freshly ground black pepper
- ✓ Nonstick cooking spray

DIRECTIONS:

- ➢ Place a large, rimmed baking sheet in the oven
- ➢ Preheat the oven to 400°F (205°C) with the pan inside.
- ➢ In a large bowl, mix the eggs and milk
- ➢ Use a fork, add the fish strips to the egg mixture and stir gently to coat
- ➢ Put the cornmeal, bread crumbs
- ➢ Add smoked paprika, salt, and pepper in a quart-size zip-top plastic bag
- ➢ Use a fork or tongs, transfer the fish to the bag
- ➢ Let the excess egg wash drip off into the bowl before transferring
- ➢ Seal the bag and shake gently to completely coat each fish stick.
- ➢ With oven mitts, carefully remove the hot baking sheet from the oven
- ➢ Spray it with nonstick cooking spray
- ➢ Use a fork or tongs, remove the fish sticks from the bag
- ➢ Arrange them on the hot baking sheet, with space between them
- ➢ (So the hot air can circulate and crisp them up)
- ➢ Bake for 5 to 8 minutes
- ➢ (Until gentle pressure with a fork causes the fish to flake)
- ➢ Serve.

NUTRITION INFORMATION: Calories: 238 fat: 2g protein: 22g carbs: 28g fiber: 1g sodium: 494mg

153 SICILIAN TUNA AND VEGGIE BOWL

Servings: 6   **Cook Time: 16 Min**   **Prep Time 10 Min**

INGREDIENTS:

- ✓ 1 pound (454 g) kale, chopped, center ribs removed
- ✓ 3 tablespoons extra-virgin olive oil
- ✓ 1 cup chopped onion
- ✓ 3 garlic cloves, minced
- ✓ 1 (2¼-ounce / 64-g) can sliced olives, drained
- ✓ ¼ cup capers
- ✓ ¼ teaspoon crushed red pepper
- ✓ 2 teaspoons sugar
- ✓ 2 (6-ounce / 170-g) cans tuna in olive oil, undrained
- ✓ 1 (15-ounce / 425-g) can cannellini beans or great northern beans, drained and rinsed
- ✓ ¼ teaspoon freshly ground black pepper
- ✓ ¼ teaspoon kosher or sea salt

DIRECTIONS:

- ➢ Fill a large stockpot three-quarters full of water, and bring to a boil
- ➢ Add the kale and cook for 2 minutes
- ➢ (This is to make the kale less bitter.)
- ➢ Drain the kale in a colander and set aside.
- ➢ Set the empty pot back on the stove over medium heat
- ➢ Pour in the oil. Add the onion and cook for 4 minutes, stirring often
- ➢ Then the garlic and cook for 1 minute, stirring often
- ➢ Join also the olives, capers, and crushed red pepper
- ➢ Cook for 1 minute, stirring often. Add the partially cooked kale and sugar
- ➢ Stir until the kale is completely coated with oil
- ➢ Cover the pot and cook for 8 minutes.
- ➢ Remove the kale from the heat, mix in the tuna, beans, pepper, and salt
- ➢ Serve.

NUTRITION INFORMATION: Calories: 372 | fat: 28g | protein: 8g | carbs: 22g | fiber: 7g | sodium: 452mg:

154 OREGANO SHRIMP PUTTANESCA

Servings: 4 **Cook Time: 9 Min** **Prep Time 10 Min**

INGREDIENTS:

- ✓ 2 tablespoons extra-virgin olive oil
- ✓ 3 anchovy fillets, drained and chopped, or 1½ teaspoons anchovy paste
- ✓ 3 garlic cloves, minced
- ✓ ½ teaspoon crushed red pepper
- ✓ 1 (14½-ounce / 411-g) can low-sodium or no-salt-added diced tomatoes, undrained
- ✓ 1 (2¼-ounce / 64-g) can sliced black olives, drained
- ✓ 2 tablespoons capers
- ✓ 1 tablespoon chopped fresh oregano or
- ✓ 1 teaspoon dried oregano
- ✓ 1 pound fresh raw shrimp (or frozen and thawed shrimp), shells and tails removed

DIRECTIONS:

- ➢ In a large skillet over medium heat, heat the oil
- ➢ Mix in the anchovies, garlic, and crushed red pepper
- ➢ Cook for 3 minutes, stirring frequently and mashing up the anchovies with a wooden spoon
- ➢ (Until they have melted into the oil)
- ➢ Stir in the tomatoes with their juices, olives, capers, and oregano
- ➢ Turn up the heat to medium-high, and bring to a simmer.
- ➢ When the sauce is lightly bubbling, stir in the shrimp
- ➢ Reduce the heat to medium
- ➢ Cook the shrimp for 6 to 8 minutes
- ➢ (Or until they turn pink and white, stirring occasionally)
- ➢ Serve.

NUTRITION INFORMATION: Calories: 362 fat: 12g protein: 30g carbs: 31g fiber: 1g sodium: 1463mg

155 SHRIMP AND VEGGIE PITA

Servings: 4 **Cook Time: 6 Min** **Prep Time 15 Min**

INGREDIENTS:

- ✓ 1 pound (454 g) medium shrimp, peeled and deveined
- ✓ 2 tablespoons olive oil
- ✓ 1 teaspoon dried oregano
- ✓ ½ teaspoon dried thyme
- ✓ ½ teaspoon garlic powder
- ✓ ¼ teaspoon onion powder
- ✓ ½ teaspoon salt
- ✓ ¼ teaspoon black pepper
- ✓ 4 whole wheat pitas
- ✓ 4 ounces (113 g) feta cheese, crumbled
- ✓ 1 cup shredded lettuce
- ✓ 1 tomato, diced
- ✓ ¼ cup black olives, sliced
- ✓ 1 lemon

DIRECTIONS:

- ➢ Preheat the oven to 380°F (193°C).
- ➢ In a medium bowl, combine the shrimp with the olive oil, oregano
- ➢ Add thyme, garlic powder, onion powder, salt, and black pepper.
- ➢ Pour shrimp in a single layer in the air fryer basket
- ➢ Cook for 6 to 8 minutes, or until cooked through.
- ➢ Remove from the air fryer
- ➢ Divide into warmed pitas with feta, lettuce, tomato, olives
- ➢ Than squeeze of lemon.

NUTRITION INFORMATION: Calories: 395 fat: 15g protein: 26g carbs: 40g fiber: 4g sodium: 728mg

156 SEA BASS WITH ROASTED ROOT VEGGIE

Servings: 15   **Cook Time: 15 Min**   **Prep Time 10 Min**

INGREDIENTS:

- ✓ 1 carrot, diced small 1 parsnip, diced small
- ✓ 1 rutabaga, diced small
- ✓ ¼ cup olive oil
- ✓ 2 teaspoons salt, divided

- ✓ 4 sea bass fillets
- ✓ ½ teaspoon onion powder
- ✓ 2 garlic cloves, minced
- ✓ 1 lemon, sliced, plus additional wedges for serving

DIRECTIONS:

- ➤ Preheat the air fryer to 380°F (193°C).
- ➤ In a small bowl, toss the carrot, parsnip, and rutabaga with olive oil and 1 teaspoon salt.
- ➤ Lightly season the sea bass with the remaining 1 teaspoon of salt and the onion powder
- ➤ Then place it into the air fryer basket in a single layer.

- ➤ Spread the garlic over the top of each fillet, then cover with lemon slices.
- ➤ Pour the prepared vegetables into the basket around and on top of the fish
- ➤ Roast for 15 minutes.
- ➤ Serve with additional lemon wedges if desired.

NUTRITION INFORMATION: Calories: 299 fat: 15g protein: 25g carbs: 13g fiber: 2g sodium: 1232mg

157 COD FILLET WITH SWISS CHARD

Servings: 4   **Cook Time: 12 Min**   **Prep Time 10 Min**

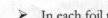

INGREDIENTS:

- ✓ 1 teaspoon salt
- ✓ ½ teaspoon dried oregano
- ✓ ½ teaspoon dried thyme
- ✓ ½ teaspoon garlic powder
- ✓ 4 cod fillets
- ✓ ½ white onion, thinly sliced
- ✓ 2 cups Swiss chard, washed, stemmed, and torn into pieces
- ✓ ¼ cup olive oil
- ✓ 1 lemon, quartered

DIRECTIONS:

- ➤ Preheat the air fryer to 380°F (193°C).
- ➤ In a small bowl, whisk together the salt, oregano, thyme, and garlic powder.
- ➤ Tear off four pieces of aluminum foil, with each sheet being large enough to envelop one cod fillet and a quarter of the vegetables.
- ➤ Place a cod fillet in the middle of each sheet of foil
- ➤ Then sprinkle on all sides with the spice mixture.

- ➤ In each foil packet, place a quarter of the onion slices and ½ cup Swiss chard
- ➤ Then drizzle 1 tablespoon olive oil and squeeze ¼ lemon over the contents of each foil packet.
- ➤ Fold and seal the sides of the foil packets
- ➤ Then place them into the air fryer basket. Steam for 12 minutes.
- ➤ Remove from the basket, and carefully open each packet to avoid a steam burn.

NUTRITION INFORMATION: Calories: 252 fat: 13g protein: 26g carbs: 4g fiber: 1g sodium: 641mg

158 POLLOCK AND VEGETABLE PITAS

Servings: 4   **Cook Time: 15 Min**   **Prep Time 10 Min**

INGREDIENTS:
- ✓ 1 pound (454 g) pollock, cut into
- ✓ 1-inch pieces
- ✓ ¼ cup olive oil
- ✓ 1 teaspoon salt
- ✓ ½ teaspoon dried oregano
- ✓ ½ teaspoon dried thyme
- ✓ ½ teaspoon garlic powder
- ✓ ¼ teaspoon cayenne 4 whole wheat pitas
- ✓ 1 cup shredded lettuce
- ✓ 2 Roma tomatoes, diced
- ✓ Nonfat plain Greek yogurt
- ✓ Lemon, quartered

DIRECTIONS:
- ➤ Preheat the air fryer to 380°F (193°C).
- ➤ In a medium bowl, combine the pollock with olive oil, salt, oregano, thyme, garlic powder, and cayenne.
- ➤ Put the pollock into the air fryer basket and cook for 15 minutes.
- ➤ Serve inside pitas with lettuce, tomato, and Greek yogurt with a lemon wedge on the side.

NUTRITION INFORMATION: Calories: 368 fat: 1g protein: 21g carbs: 38g fiber: 5g sodium: 514mg

159 DILL AND GARLIC STUFFED RED SNAPPER

Servings: 4   **Cook Time: 35 Min**   **Prep Time 10 Min**

INGREDIENTS:
- ✓ 1 teaspoon salt
- ✓ ½ teaspoon black pepper
- ✓ ½ teaspoon ground cumin
- ✓ ¼ teaspoon cayenne
- ✓ 1 (1- to 1½-pound / 454- to 680-g) whole red snapper, cleaned and patted dry
- ✓ 2 tablespoons olive oil
- ✓ 2 garlic cloves, minced
- ✓ ¼ cup fresh dill
- ✓ Lemon wedges, for serving

DIRECTIONS:
- ➤ Preheat the air fryer to 360°F (182°C)
- ➤ In a small bowl, mix together the salt, pepper, cumin, and cayenne.
- ➤ Coat the outside of the fish with olive oil
- ➤ Then sprinkle the seasoning blend over the outside of the fish
- ➤ Stuff the minced garlic and dill inside the cavity of the fish.
- ➤ Place the snapper into the basket of the air fryer and roast for 20 minutes
- ➤ Flip the snapper over, and roast for 15 minutes more
- ➤ (Or until the snapper reaches an internal temperature of 145°F (63°C))

NUTRITION INFORMATION: Calories: 125 fat: 1g protein: 23g carbs: 2g fiber: 0g sodium: 562mg

160 EASY TUNA STEAKS

Servings: 4 **Cook Time: 8 Min** **Prep Time 10 Min**

INGREDIENTS:

- ✓ 1 teaspoon garlic powder
- ✓ ½ teaspoon salt
- ✓ ¼ teaspoon dried thyme
- ✓ ¼ teaspoon dried oregano

- ✓ 4 tuna steaks
- ✓ 2 tablespoons olive oil
- ✓ 1 lemon, quartered

DIRECTIONS:

- ➢ Preheat the air fryer to 380°F (193°C).
- ➢ In a small bowl, whisk together the garlic powder, salt, thyme, and oregano.
- ➢ Coat the tuna steaks with olive oil
- ➢ Season both sides of each steak with the seasoning blend

- ➢ Place the steaks in a single layer in the air fryer basket.
- ➢ Cook for 5 minutes, then flip and cook for an additional 3 to 4 minutes.

NUTRITION INFORMATION: Calories: 269 fat: 13g protein: 33g carbs: 1g fiber: 0g sodium: 231mg

161 GREEK-STYLE LAMB BURGERS

Servings: 4 **Cook Time: 10 Min** **Prep Time 10 Min**

INGREDIENTS:

- ✓ 1 pound (454 g) ground lamb
- ✓ ½ teaspoon salt
- ✓ ½ teaspoon freshly ground black pepper
- ✓ 4 tablespoons feta cheese, crumbled
- ✓ Buns, toppings, and tzatziki, for serving (optional)

DIRECTIONS:

- ➢ Preheat a grill, grill pan, or lightly oiled skillet to high heat.
- ➢ In a large bowl, using your hands
- ➢ Combine the lamb with the salt and pepper.
- ➢ Divide the meat into 4 portions. Divide each portion in half to make a top and a bottom
- ➢ Flatten each half into a 3-inch circle
- ➢ Make a dent in the center of one of the halves and place 1 tablespoon of the feta cheese in the center
- ➢ Place the second half of the patty on top of the feta cheese
- ➢ Press down to close the 2 halves together, making it resemble a round burger.
- ➢ Cook the stuffed patty for 3 minutes on each side, for medium-well
- ➢ Serve on a bun with your favorite toppings and tzatziki sauce, if desired.

NUTRITION INFORMATION: Calories: 345 fat: 29g protein: 20g carbs: 1g fiber: 0g sodium: 462mg

162 BRAISED VEAL SHANKS

Servings: 4   **Cook Time: 2 H**   **Prep Time 10 Min**

INGREDIENTS:

- ✓ 4 veal shanks, bone in
- ✓ ½ cup flour
- ✓ 4 tablespoons extra-virgin olive oil
- ✓ 1 large onion, chopped
- ✓ 5 cloves garlic, sliced
- ✓ 2 teaspoons salt
- ✓ 1 tablespoon fresh thyme
- ✓ 3 tablespoons tomato paste
- ✓ 6 cups water
- ✓ Cooked noodles, for serving (optional)

DIRECTIONS:

- ➤ Preheat the oven to 350°F (180°C).
- ➤ Dredge the veal shanks in the flour.
- ➤ Pour the olive oil into a large oven-safe pot or pan over medium heat
- ➤ Add the veal shanks
- ➤ Brown the veal on both sides, about 4 minutes each side
- ➤ Remove the veal from pot and set aside.
- ➤ Add the onion, garlic, salt, thyme, and tomato paste to the pan
- ➤ Cook for 3 to 4 minutes. Add the water, and stir to combine.
- ➤ Then the veal back to the pan, and bring to a simmer
- ➤ Cover the pan with a lid or foil and bake for 1 hour and 50 minutes
- ➤ Remove from the oven and serve with cooked noodles, if desired.

NUTRITION INFORMATION: Calories: 400 fat: 19g protein: 39g carbs: 18g fiber: 2g sodium: 1368mg

163 GRILLED BEEF KEBABS

Servings: 6   **Cook Time: 10 Min**   **Prep Time 15 Min**

INGREDIENTS:

- ✓ 2 pounds (907 g) beef fillet
- ✓ 1½ teaspoons salt
- ✓ 1 teaspoon freshly ground black pepper
- ✓ ½ teaspoon ground allspice
- ✓ ½ teaspoon ground nutmeg
- ✓ ⅓ cup extra-virgin olive oil
- ✓ 1 large onion, cut into
- ✓ 8 quarters
- ✓ 1 large red bell pepper, cut into
- ✓ 1-inch cubes

DIRECTIONS:

- ➤ Preheat a grill, grill pan, or lightly oiled skillet to high heat.
- ➤ Cut the beef into 1-inch cubes and put them in a large bowl.
- ➤ In a small bowl, mix together the salt, black pepper, allspice, and nutmeg.
- ➤ Pour the olive oil over the beef and toss to coat the beef
- ➤ Then evenly sprinkle the seasoning over the beef and toss to coat all pieces.
- ➤ Skewer the beef, alternating every 1 or 2 pieces with a piece of onion or bell pepper.
- ➤ To cook, place the skewers on the grill or skillet, and turn every 2 to 3 minutes until all sides have cooked to desired
- ➤ (Doneness, 6 minutes for medium-rare, 8 minutes for well done)
- ➤ Serve warm.

NUTRITION INFORMATION: Calories: 485 fat: 36g protein: 35g carbs: 4g fiber: 1g sodium: 1453mg

164 MEDITERRANEAN GRILLED SKIRT STEAK

Servings: 4 **Cook Time: 10 Min** **Prep Time 10 Min**

INGREDIENTS:
- ✓ 1 pound (454 g) skirt steak
- ✓ 1 teaspoon salt
- ✓ ½ teaspoon freshly ground black pepper
- ✓ 2 cups prepared hummus
- ✓ 1 tablespoon extra-virgin olive oil
- ✓ ½ cup pine nuts

DIRECTIONS:
- ➤ Preheat a grill, grill pan, or lightly oiled skillet to medium heat.
- ➤ Season both sides of the steak with salt and pepper.
- ➤ Cook the meat on each side for 3 to 5 minutes; 3 minutes for medium, and 5 minutes on each side for well done
- ➤ Let the meat rest for 5 minutes.
- ➤ Slice the meat into thin strips.
- ➤ Spread the hummus on a serving dish, and evenly distribute the beef on top of the hummus.
- ➤ In a small saucepan, over low heat, add the olive oil and pine nuts
- ➤ Toast them for 3 minutes, constantly stirring them with a spoon so that they don't burn.
- ➤ Spoon the pine nuts over the beef and serve.

NUTRITION INFORMATION: Calories: 602 fat: 41g protein: 42g carbs: 20g fiber: 8g sodium: 1141mg

165 BEEF KEFTA

Servings: 4 **Cook Time: 5 Min** **Prep Time 10 Min**

INGREDIENTS:
- ✓ 1 medium onion
- ✓ ⅓ cup fresh Italian parsley
- ✓ 1 pound (454 g) ground beef

- ✓ ¼ teaspoon ground cumin
- ✓ ¼ teaspoon cinnamon
- ✓ 1 teaspoon salt
- ✓ ½ teaspoon freshly ground black pepper

DIRECTIONS:
- ➤ Preheat a grill or grill pan to high.
- ➤ Mince the onion and parsley in a food processor until finely chopped.
- ➤ In a large bowl, using your hands
- ➤ Combine the beef with the onion mix, ground cumin, cinnamon, salt, and pepper.

- ➤ Divide the meat into 6 portions. Form each portion into a flat oval.
- ➤ Place the patties on the grill or grill pan and cook for 3 minutes on each side.

NUTRITION INFORMATION: Calories: 203 fat: 10g protein: 24g carbs: 3g fiber: 1g sodium: 655mg

166 BEEF AND POTATOES WITH TAHINI SAUCE

Servings: 6   **Cook Time: 30 Min**   **Prep Time 10 Min**

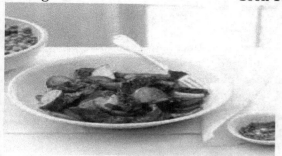

INGREDIENTS:
- ✓ 1 pound (454 g) ground beef
- ✓ 2 teaspoons salt, divided
- ✓ ½ teaspoon freshly ground black pepper
- ✓ 1 large onion, finely chopped
- ✓ 10 medium golden potatoes
- ✓ 2 tablespoons extra-virgin olive oil
- ✓ 3 cups Greek yogurt
- ✓ 1 cup tahini
- ✓ 3 cloves garlic, minced 2 cups water

DIRECTIONS:
- ➤ Preheat the oven to 450°F (235°C).
- ➤ In a large bowl, using your hands, combine the beef with 1 teaspoon salt, black pepper, and the onion.
- ➤ Form meatballs of medium size (about 1-inch), using about 2 tablespoons of the beef mixture
- ➤ Place them in a deep 8-by-8-inch casserole dish.
- ➤ Cut the potatoes into ¼-inch-thick slices
- ➤ Toss them with the olive oil.
- ➤ Lay the potato slices flat on a lined baking sheet.
- ➤ Put the baking sheet with the potatoes and the casserole dish with the meatballs in the oven
- ➤ Bake for 20 minutes.
- ➤ In a large bowl, mix together the yogurt, tahini, garlic, remaining 1 teaspoon salt, and water; set aside.

- ➤ Once you take the meatballs and potatoes out of the oven
- ➤ Use a spatula to transfer the potatoes from the baking sheet to the casserole dish with the meatballs
- ➤ Leave the beef drippings in the casserole dish for added flavor.
- ➤ Reduce the oven temperature to 375°F (190°C)
- ➤ Pour the yogurt tahini sauce over the beef and potatoes
- ➤ Return it to the oven for 10 minutes
- ➤ Once baking is complete, serve warm with a side of rice or pita bread.

NUTRITION INFORMATION: Calories: 1078 fat: 59g protein: 58g carbs: 89g fiber: 11g sodium: 1368mg

167 MEDITERRANEAN LAMB BOWLS

Servings: 2   **Cook Time: 15 Min**   **Prep Time 15 Min**

INGREDIENTS:
- ✓ 2 tablespoons extra-virgin olive oil
- ✓ ¼ cup diced yellow onion
- ✓ 1 pound (454 g) ground lamb
- ✓ 1 teaspoon dried mint
- ✓ 1 teaspoon dried parsley
- ✓ ½ teaspoon red pepper flakes
- ✓ ¼ teaspoon garlic powder

- ✓ 1 cup cooked rice
- ✓ ½ teaspoon za'atar seasoning
- ✓ ½ cup halved cherry tomatoes
- ✓ 1 cucumber, peeled and diced
- ✓ 1 cup store-bought hummus
- ✓ 1 cup crumbled feta cheese
- ✓ 2 pita breads, warmed (optional)

DIRECTIONS:
- ➤ In a large sauté pan or skillet, heat the olive oil over medium heat
- ➤ Cook the onion for about 2 minutes, until fragrant
- ➤ Add the lamb and mix well, breaking up the meat as you cook
- ➤ Once the lamb is halfway cooked, add mint, parsley, red pepper flakes, and garlic powder.

- ➤ In a medium bowl, mix together the cooked rice and za'atar
- ➤ Then divide between individual serving bowls
- ➤ Join also the seasoned lamb
- ➤ Then top the bowls with the tomatoes, cucumber, hummus, feta, and pita (if using).

NUTRITION INFORMATION: Calories: 1312 fat: 96g protein: 62g carbs: 62g fiber: 12g sodium: 1454mg

168 BRAISED GARLIC FLANK STEAK WITH ARTICHOKES

Servings: 6   **Cook Time: 60 Min**   **Prep Time 15 Min**

INGREDIENTS:

- ✓ 4 tablespoons grapeseed oil, divided
- ✓ 2 pounds (907 g) flank steak
- ✓ 1 (14-ounce / 397-g) can artichoke hearts, drained and roughly chopped
- ✓ 1 onion, diced
- ✓ 8 garlic cloves, chopped
- ✓ 1 (32-ounce / 907-g) container low-sodium beef broth
- ✓ 1 (14½-ounce / 411-g) can diced tomatoes, drained
- ✓ 1 cup tomato sauce
- ✓ 2 tablespoons tomato paste
- ✓ 1 teaspoon dried oregano
- ✓ 1 teaspoon dried parsley
- ✓ 1 teaspoon dried basil
- ✓ ½ teaspoon ground cumin
- ✓ 3 bay leaves
- ✓ 2 to 3 cups cooked couscous (optional)

DIRECTIONS:

- ➢ Preheat the oven to 450°F (235°C).
- ➢ In an oven-safe sauté pan or skillet, heat 3 tablespoons of oil on medium heat
- ➢ Sear the steak for 2 minutes per side on both sides
- ➢ Transfer the steak to the oven for 30 minutes, or until desired tenderness.
- ➢ Meanwhile, in a large pot, combine the remaining 1 tablespoon of oil, artichoke hearts, onion, and garlic
- ➢ Pour in the beef broth, tomatoes, tomato sauce, and tomato paste
- ➢ Stir in oregano, parsley, basil, cumin, and bay leaves.
- ➢ Cook the vegetables, covered, for 30 minutes
- ➢ Remove bay leaf and serve with flank steak and ½ cup of couscous per plate, if using.

NUTRITION INFORMATION: Calories: 577 fat: 28g protein: 55g carbs: 22g fiber: 6g sodium: 1405mg

169 TRADITIONAL CHICKEN SHAWARMA

Servings: 6   **Cook Time: 15 Min**   **Prep Time 15 Min**

INGREDIENTS:

- ✓ 2 pounds (907 g) boneless and skinless chicken
- ✓ ½ cup lemon juice
- ✓ ½ cup extra-virgin olive oil
- ✓ 3 tablespoons minced garlic
- ✓ 1½ teaspoons salt
- ✓ ½ teaspoon freshly ground black pepper
- ✓ ½ teaspoon ground cardamom
- ✓ ½ teaspoon cinnamon
- ✓ Hummus and pita bread, for serving (optional)

DIRECTIONS:

- ➢ Cut the chicken into ¼-inch strips and put them into a large bowl.
- ➢ In a separate bowl, whisk together the lemon juice, olive oil
- ➢ Then garlic, salt, pepper, cardamom, and cinnamon.
- ➢ Pour the dressing over the chicken and stir to coat all of the chicken.
- ➢ Let the chicken sit for about 10 minutes.
- ➢ Heat a large pan over medium-high heat
- ➢ Cook the chicken pieces for 12 minutes, using tongs to turn the chicken over every few minutes.
- ➢ Serve with hummus and pita bread, if desired.

NUTRITION INFORMATION: Calories: 477 | fat: 32g | protein: 47g | carbs: 5g | fiber: 1g | sodium: 1234mg

170 CHICKEN SHISH TAWOOK

Servings: 6 **Cook Time: 15 Min** **Prep Time 15 Min**

INGREDIENTS:

- ✓ 2 tablespoons garlic, minced
- ✓ 2 tablespoons tomato paste
- ✓ 1 teaspoon smoked paprika
- ✓ ½ cup lemon juice
- ✓ ½ cup extra-virgin olive oil
- ✓ 1½ teaspoons salt
- ✓ ½ teaspoon freshly ground black pepper
- ✓ 2 pounds (907 g) boneless and skinless chicken (breasts or thighs)
- ✓ Rice, tzatziki, or hummus, for serving (optional)

DIRECTIONS:

- ➤ In a large bowl, add the garlic, tomato paste, paprika,
- ➤ Then lemon juice, olive oil, salt, and pepper and whisk to combine.
- ➤ Cut the chicken into ½-inch cubes
- ➤ Put them into the bowl; toss to coat with the marinade
- ➤ Set aside for at least 10 minutes.
- ➤ To grill, preheat the grill on high
- ➤ Thread the chicken onto skewers
- ➤ Cook for 3 minutes per side, for a total of 9 minutes.
- ➤ To cook in a pan, preheat the pan on high heat
- ➤ Add the chicken, and cook for 9 minutes, turning over the chicken using tongs.
- ➤ Serve the chicken with rice, tzatziki, or hummus, if desired.

NUTRITION INFORMATION: Calories: 482 fat: 32g protein: 47g carbs: 6g fiber: 1g sodium: 1298mg

171 LEMON-GARLIC WHOLE CHICKEN AND POTATOES

Servings: 6 **Cook Time: 45 Min** **Prep Time 10 Min**

INGREDIENTS:

- ✓ 1 cup garlic, minced
- ✓ 1½ cups lemon juice
- ✓ 1 cup plus
- ✓ 2 tablespoons extra-virgin olive oil, divided
- ✓ 1½ teaspoons salt, divided
- ✓ 1 teaspoon freshly ground black pepper
- ✓ 1 whole chicken, cut into
- ✓ 8 pieces
- ✓ 1 pound (454 g) fingerling or red potatoes

DIRECTIONS:

- ➤ Preheat the oven to 400°F (205°C).
- ➤ In a large bowl, whisk together the garlic, lemon juice, 1 cup of olive oil, 1 teaspoon of salt, and pepper.
- ➤ Put the chicken in a large baking dish and pour half of the lemon sauce over the chicken
- ➤ Cover the baking dish with foil, and cook for 20 minutes.
- ➤ Cut the potatoes in half, and toss to coat with 2 tablespoons olive oil and 1 teaspoon of salt
- ➤ Put them on a baking sheet and bake for 20 minutes in the same oven as the chicken.
- ➤ Take both the chicken and potatoes out of the oven
- ➤ Use a spatula, transfer the potatoes to the baking dish with the chicken
- ➤ Pour the remaining sauce over the potatoes and chicken
- ➤ Bake for another 25 minutes.
- ➤ Transfer the chicken and potatoes to a serving dish
- ➤ Spoon the garlic- lemon sauce from the pan on top.

NUTRITION INFORMATION: Calories: 959 fat: 78g protein: 33g carbs: 37g fiber: 4g sodium: 1005mg

172 LEMON CHICKEN THIGHS WITH VEGETABLES

Servings: 4   **Cook Time: 45 Min**   **Prep Time 15 Min**

INGREDIENTS:

- ✓ 6 tablespoons extra-virgin olive oil, divided
- ✓ 4 large garlic cloves, crushed
- ✓ 1 tablespoon dried basil
- ✓ 1 tablespoon dried parsley
- ✓ 1 tablespoon salt
- ✓ ½ tablespoon thyme
- ✓ 4 skin-on, bone-in chicken thighs

- ✓ 6 medium portobello mushrooms, quartered
- ✓ 1 large zucchini, sliced
- ✓ 1 large carrot, thinly sliced
- ✓ ⅛ cup pitted Kalamata olives
- ✓ 8 pieces sun-dried tomatoes (optional)
- ✓ ½ cup dry white wine
- ✓ 1 lemon, sliced

DIRECTIONS:

- ➤ In a small bowl, combine 4 tablespoons of olive oil, the garlic cloves, basil, parsley, salt, and thyme
- ➤ Store half of the marinade in a jar and, in a bowl
- ➤ Combine the remaining half to marinate the chicken thighs for about 30 minutes.
- ➤ Preheat the oven to 425°F (220°C).
- ➤ In a large skillet or oven-safe pan, heat the remaining 2 tablespoons of olive oil over medium-high heat
- ➤ Sear the chicken for 3 to 5 minutes on each side until golden brown, and set aside.

- ➤ In the same pan, sauté portobello mushrooms, zucchini, and carrot for about 5 minutes
- ➤ (Or until lightly browned)
- ➤ Add the chicken thighs, olives, and sun-dried tomatoes (if using)
- ➤ Pour the wine over the chicken thighs.
- ➤ Cover the pan and cook for about 10 minutes over medium-low heat.
- ➤ Uncover the pan and transfer it to the oven
- ➤ Cook for 15 more minutes, or until the chicken skin is crispy and the juices run clear
- ➤ Top with lemon slices.

NUTRITION INFORMATION: Calories: 544 fat: 41g protein: 28g carbs: 20g fiber: 11g sodium: 1848mg

173 YOGURT-MARINATED CHICKEN

Servings: 2   **Cook Time: 30 Min**   **Prep Time 15 Min**

INGREDIENTS:

- ✓ ½ cup plain Greek yogurt 3 garlic cloves, minced
- ✓ 2 tablespoons minced fresh oregano (or 1 tablespoon dried oregano)
- ✓ Zest of 1 lemon

- ✓ 1 tablespoon olive oil
- ✓ ½ teaspoon salt
- ✓ 2 (4-ounce / 113-g) boneless, skinless chicken breasts

DIRECTIONS:

- ➤ In a medium bowl, add the yogurt, garlic, oregano, lemon zest, olive oil, and salt and stir to combine
- ➤ If the yogurt is very thick, you may need to add a few tablespoons of water or a squeeze of lemon juice to thin it a bit.
- ➤ Add the chicken to the bowl
- ➤ Toss it in the marinade to coat it well

- ➤ Cover and refrigerate the chicken for at least 30 minutes or up to overnight.
- ➤ Preheat the oven to 350°F (180°C) and set the rack to the middle position.
- ➤ Place the chicken in a baking dish and roast for 30 minutes
- ➤ (Or until chicken reaches an internal temperature of 165°F (74°C))

NUTRITION INFORMATION: Calories: 255 fat: 13g protein: 29g carbs: 8g fiber: 2g sodium: 694mg

174 FETA STUFFED CHICKEN BREASTS

Servings: 4 **Cook Time: 20 Min** **Prep Time 10 Min**

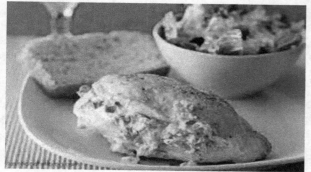

INGREDIENTS:
- ✓ ⅓ cup cooked brown rice
- ✓ 1 teaspoon shawarma seasoning
- ✓ 4 (6-ounce / 170-g) boneless skinless chicken breasts
- ✓ 1 tablespoon harissa
- ✓ 3 tablespoons extra-virgin olive oil, divided
- ✓ Salt and freshly ground black pepper, to taste
- ✓ 4 small dried apricots, halved
- ✓ ⅓ cup crumbled feta
- ✓ 1 tablespoon chopped fresh parsley

DIRECTIONS:
- ➤ Preheat the oven to 375°F (190°C).
- ➤ In a medium bowl, mix the rice and shawarma seasoning and set aside.
- ➤ Butterfly the chicken breasts by slicing them almost in half
- ➤ Start at the thickest part and folding them open like a book.
- ➤ In a small bowl, mix the harissa with 1 tablespoon of olive oil
- ➤ Brush the chicken with the harissa oil and season with salt and pepper
- ➤ The harissa adds a nice heat, so feel free to add a thicker coating for more spice.

- ➤ Onto one side of each chicken breast, spoon 1 to 2 tablespoons of rice
- ➤ Then layer 2 apricot halves in each breast
- ➤ Divide the feta between the chicken breasts and fold the other side over the filling to close.
- ➤ In an oven-safe sauté pan or skillet, heat the remaining 2 tablespoons of olive oil
- ➤ Sear the breast for 2 minutes on each side
- ➤ Then place the pan into the oven for 15 minutes, or until fully cooked and juices run clear
- ➤ Serve, garnished with parsley.

NUTRITION INFORMATION: Calories: 321 fat: 17g protein: 37g carbs: 8g fiber: 1g sodium: 410mg

175 CHICKEN SAUSAGE AND TOMATO WITH FARRO

Servings: 2 **Cook Time: 45 Min** **Prep Time 10 Min**

INGREDIENTS:
- ✓ 1 tablespoon olive oil
- ✓ ½ medium onion, diced
- ✓ ¼ cup julienned sun-dried tomatoes packed in olive oil and herbs
- ✓ 8 ounces (227 g) hot Italian chicken sausage, removed from the casing

- ✓ ¾ cup farro
- ✓ 1½ cups low-sodium chicken stock
- ✓ 2 cups loosely packed arugula
- ✓ 4 to 5 large fresh basil leaves, sliced thin
- ✓ Salt, to taste

DIRECTIONS:
- ➤ Heat the olive oil in a sauté pan over medium-high heat
- ➤ Add the onion and sauté for 5 minutes
- ➤ Then the sun-dried tomatoes and chicken sausage
- ➤ Stir to break up the sausage
- ➤ Cook for 7 minutes, or until the sausage is no longer pink.
- ➤ Stir in the farro. Let it toast for 3 minutes, stirring occasionally.

- ➤ Join also the chicken stock and bring the mixture to a boil
- ➤ Cover the pan and reduce the heat to medium-low
- ➤ Let it simmer for 30 minutes, or until the farro is tender.
- ➤ Stir in the arugula and let it wilt slightly
- ➤ Add the basil, and season with salt.

NUTRITION INFORMATION: Calories: 491 fat: 18g protein: 31g carbs: 53g fiber: 6g sodium: 765mg

176 CHICKEN, MUSHROOMS, AND TARRAGON PASTA

Servings: 2 **Cook Time: 15 Min** **Prep Time 15 Min**

INGREDIENTS:
- ✓ 2 tablespoons olive oil, divided
- ✓ ½ medium onion, minced
- ✓ 4 ounces (113 g) baby bella (cremini) mushrooms, sliced
- ✓ 2 small garlic cloves, minced
- ✓ 8 ounces (227 g) chicken cutlets
- ✓ 2 teaspoons tomato paste
- ✓ 2 teaspoons dried tarragon
- ✓ 2 cups low-sodium chicken stock 6 ounces (170 g) pappardelle pasta
- ✓ ¼ cup plain full-fat Greek yogurt
- ✓ Salt, to taste
- ✓ Freshly ground black pepper, to taste

DIRECTIONS:
- ➤ Heat 1 tablespoon of the olive oil in a sauté pan over medium-high heat
- ➤ Add the onion and mushrooms and sauté for 5 minutes
- ➤ Then the garlic and cook for 1 minute more.
- ➤ Move the vegetables to the edges of the pan
- ➤ Add the remaining 1 tablespoon of olive oil to the center of the pan
- ➤ Place the cutlets in the center and let them cook for about 3 minutes
- ➤ (Or until they lift up easily and are golden brown on the bottom)
- ➤ Flip the chicken and cook for another 3 minutes.
- ➤ Mix in the tomato paste and tarragon
- ➤ Then the chicken stock and stir well to combine everything
- ➤ Bring the stock to a boil.
- ➤ Add the pappardelle
- ➤ Break up the pasta if needed to fit into the pan
- ➤ Stir the noodles so they don't stick to the bottom of the pan.
- ➤ Cover the sauté pan and reduce the heat to medium-low
- ➤ Let the chicken and noodles simmer for 15 minutes, stirring occasionally
- ➤ (Until the pasta is cooked and the liquid is mostly absorbed)
- ➤ If the liquid absorbs too quickly and the pasta isn't cooked, add more water or chicken stock, about ¼ cup at a time as needed.
- ➤ Remove the pan from the heat.
- ➤ Stir 2 tablespoons of the hot liquid from the pan into the yogurt
- ➤ Pour the tempered yogurt into the pan
- ➤ Stir well to mix it into the sauce. Season with salt and pepper.
- ➤ The sauce will tighten up as it cools, so if it seems too thick, add a few tablespoons of water.

NUTRITION INFORMATION: Calories: 556 | fat: 17g | protein: 42g | carbs: 56g | fiber: 1g | sodium: 190mg

177 POACHED CHICKEN BREAST WITH ROMESCO SAUCE

Servings: 6   **Cook Time: 12 Min**   **Prep Time 10 Min**

INGREDIENTS:

- ✓ 1½ pounds (680 g) boneless, skinless chicken breasts, cut into 6 pieces
- ✓ 1 carrot, halved
- ✓ 1 celery stalk, halved
- ✓ ½ onion, halved
- ✓ 2 garlic cloves, smashed
- ✓ 3 sprigs fresh thyme or rosemary
- ✓ 1 cup romesco sauce
- ✓ 2 tablespoons chopped fresh flat-leaf (Italian) parsley
- ✓ ¼ teaspoon freshly ground black pepper

DIRECTIONS:

- ➤ Put the chicken in a medium saucepan
- ➤ Fill with water until there's about one inch of liquid above the chicken
- ➤ Add the carrot, celery, onion, garlic, and thyme
- ➤ Cover and bring it to a boil
- ➤ Reduce the heat to low (keeping it covered), and cook for 12 to 15 minutes
- ➤ (Or until the internal temperature of the chicken measures 165°F (74°C) on a meat thermometer and any juices run clear)
- ➤ Remove the chicken from the water and let sit for 5 minutes.
- ➤ When you're ready to serve
- ➤ Spread ¾ cup of romesco sauce on the bottom of a serving platter
- ➤ Arrange the chicken breasts on top
- ➤ Drizzle with the remaining romesco sauce
- ➤ Sprinkle the tops with parsley and pepper.

NUTRITION INFORMATION: Calories: 270 fat: 10g protein: 13g carbs: 31g fiber: 2g sodium: 647mg

178 TAHINI CHICKEN RICE BOWLS WITH APRICOTS

Servings: 4   **Cook Time: 15 Min**   **Prep Time 15 Min**

INGREDIENTS:

- ✓ 1 cup uncooked instant brown rice
- ✓ ¼ cup tahini or peanut butter (tahini for nut-free)
- ✓ ¼ cup 2% plain Greek yogurt
- ✓ 2 tablespoons chopped scallions, green and white parts
- ✓ 1 tablespoon freshly squeezed lemon juice
- ✓ 1 tablespoon water
- ✓ 1 teaspoon ground cumin
- ✓ ¾ teaspoon ground cinnamon
- ✓ ¼ teaspoon kosher or sea salt
- ✓ 2 cups chopped cooked chicken breast
- ✓ ½ cup chopped dried apricots
- ✓ 2 cups peeled and chopped seedless cucumber
- ✓ 4 teaspoons sesame seeds
- ✓ Fresh mint leaves, for serving (optional)

DIRECTIONS:

- ➤ Cook the brown rice according to the package instructions.
- ➤ While the rice is cooking, in a medium bowl
- ➤ Mix together the tahini, yogurt, scallions, lemon juice, water, cumin, cinnamon, and salt
- ➤ Transfer half the tahini mixture to another medium bowl
- ➤ Mix the chicken into the first bowl.
- ➤ When the rice is done, mix it into the second bowl of tahini
- ➤ (The one without the chicken).
- ➤ To assemble, divide the chicken among four bowls
- ➤ Spoon the rice mixture next to the chicken in each bowl
- ➤ Next to the chicken, place the dried apricots, and in the remaining empty section, add the cucumbers
- ➤ Sprinkle with sesame seeds, and top with mint, if desired, and serve.

NUTRITION INFORMATION: Calories: 335 fat: 10g protein: 31g carbs: 30g fiber: 3g sodium: 345mg

179 ROASTED ARTICHOKES WITH CHICKEN THIGH

Servings: 4   **Cook Time: 20 Min**   **Prep Time 5 Min**

INGREDIENTS:

- ✓ 2 large lemons
- ✓ 3 tablespoons extra-virgin olive oil, divided
- ✓ ½ teaspoon kosher or sea salt
- ✓ 2 large artichokes
- ✓ 4 (6-ounce / 170-g) bone-in, skin-on chicken thighs

DIRECTIONS:

- ➢ Put a large, rimmed baking sheet in the oven
- ➢ Preheat the oven to 450°F (235°C) with the pan inside
- ➢ Tear off four sheets of aluminum foil about 8-by-10 inches each; set aside.
- ➢ Use a Microplane or citrus zester, zest 1 lemon into a large bowl
- ➢ Halve both lemons and squeeze all the juice into the bowl with the zest
- ➢ Whisk in 2 tablespoons of oil and the salt. Set aside.
- ➢ Rinse the artichokes with cool water, and dry with a clean towel
- ➢ Use a sharp knife, cut about 1½ inches off the tip of each artichoke
- ➢ Cut about ¼ inch off each stem
- ➢ Halve each artichoke lengthwise so each piece has equal amounts of stem
- ➢ Immediately plunge the artichoke halves into the lemon juice and oil mixture (To prevent browning)
- ➢ Turn to coat on all sides
- ➢ Lay one artichoke half flat-side down in the center of a sheet of aluminum foil
- ➢ Close up loosely to make a foil packet
- ➢ Repeat the process with the remaining three artichoke halves. Set the packets aside.
- ➢ Put the chicken in the remaining lemon juice mixture and turn to coat
- ➢ Use oven mitts, carefully remove the hot baking sheet from the oven
- ➢ Pour on the remaining tablespoon of oil; tilt the pan to coat
- ➢ Carefully arrange the chicken, skin-side down, on the hot baking sheet
- ➢ Place the artichoke packets, flat-side down, on the baking sheet as well
- ➢ (Arrange the artichoke packets and chicken with space between them so air can circulate around them.)
- ➢ Roast for 20 minutes
- ➢ (Or until the internal temperature of the chicken measures 165°F (74°C) on a meat thermometer and any juices run clear)
- ➢ Before serving, check the artichokes for doneness by pulling on a leaf
- ➢ If it comes out easily, the artichoke is ready.

NUTRITION INFORMATION: Calories: 832 | fat: 79g | protein: 19g | carbs: 11g | fiber: 4g | sodium: 544mg

180 CHICKEN BREAST WITH TOMATO AND BASIL

Servings: 4   **Cook Time: 20 Min**   **Prep Time 10**

INGREDIENTS:

- ✓ Nonstick cooking spray
- ✓ 1 pound (454 g) boneless, skinless chicken breasts
- ✓ 2 tablespoons extra-virgin olive oil
- ✓ ¼ teaspoon freshly ground black pepper
- ✓ ¼ teaspoon kosher or sea salt
- ✓ 1 large tomato, sliced thinly
- ✓ 1 cup shredded Mozzarella or 4 ounces fresh Mozzarella cheese, diced
- ✓ 1 (14½-ounce / 411-g) can low-sodium or no-salt-added crushed tomatoes
- ✓ 2 tablespoons fresh torn basil leaves
- ✓ 4 teaspoons balsamic vinegar

DIRECTIONS:

- ➤ Set one oven rack about 4 inches below the broiler element
- ➤ Preheat the oven to 450°F (235°C)
- ➤ Line a large, rimmed baking sheet with aluminum foil
- ➤ Place a wire cooling rack on the aluminum foil
- ➤ Spray the rack with nonstick cooking spray. Set aside.
- ➤ Cut the chicken into 4 pieces (if they aren't already)
- ➤ Put the chicken breasts in a large zip-top plastic bag
- ➤ With a rolling pin or meat mallet, pound the chicken so it is evenly flattened, about ¼-inch thick
- ➤ Add the oil, pepper, and salt to the bag
- ➤ Reseal the bag, and massage the ingredients into the chicken
- ➤ Take the chicken out of the bag and place it on the prepared wire rack.
- ➤ Cook the chicken for 15 to 18 minutes
- ➤ (Or until the internal temperature of the chicken is 165°F (74°C) on a meat thermometer and the juices run clear)
- ➤ Turn the oven to the high broiler setting
- ➤ Layer the tomato slices on each chicken breast, and top with the Mozzarella.
- ➤ Broil the chicken for another 2 to 3 minutes
- ➤ (Or until the cheese is melted)
- ➤ (Don't let the chicken burn on the edges)
- ➤ Remove the chicken from the oven
- ➤ While the chicken is cooking, pour the crushed tomatoes into a small, microwave-safe bowl
- ➤ Cover the bowl with a paper towel, and microwave for about 1 minute on high, until hot
- ➤ When you're ready to serve, divide the tomatoes among four dinner plates
- ➤ Place each chicken breast on top of the tomatoes
- ➤ Top with the basil and a drizzle of balsamic vinegar.

NUTRITION INFORMATION: Calories: 258 fat: 9g protein: 14g carbs: 28g fiber: 3g sodium: 573mg

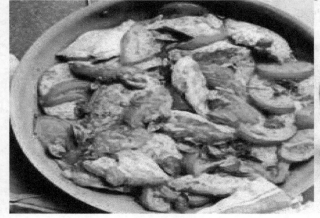

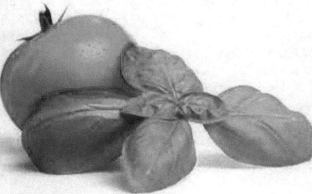

181 MASCARPONE WITH FIG CROSTINI

Servings: 8   **Cook Time: 10 Min**   **Prep Time 10 Min**

INGREDIENTS:
- ✓ 1 long French baguette
- ✓ 4 tablespoons (½ stick) salted butter, melted (optional)
- ✓ 1 (8-ounce / 227-g) tub mascarpone cheese
- ✓ 1 (12-ounce / 340-g) jar fig jam or preserves

DIRECTIONS:

- ➤ Preheat the oven to 350°F (180°C).
- ➤ Slice the bread into ¼-inch-thick slices.
- ➤ Arrange the sliced bread on a baking sheet and brush each slice with the melted butter (if desired).
- ➤ Put the baking sheet in the oven and toast the bread for 5 to 7 minutes, just until golden brown.
- ➤ Let the bread cool slightly
- ➤ Spread about a teaspoon or so of the mascarpone cheese on each piece of bread.
- ➤ Top with a teaspoon or so of the jam. Serve immediately.

NUTRITION INFORMATION: Calories: 445 fat: 24g protein: 3g carbs: 48g fiber: 5g sodium: 314mg

182 SESAME SEED COOKIES

Cookies: 16   **Cook Time: 15 Min**   **Prep Time 10 Min**

INGREDIENTS:
- ✓ 1 cup sesame seeds, hulled 1 cup sugar
- ✓ 8 tablespoons (1 stick) salted butter, softened (optional)
- ✓ 2 large eggs
- ✓ 1¼ cups flour

DIRECTIONS:

- ➤ Preheat the oven to 350°F (180°C)
- ➤ Toast the sesame seeds on a baking sheet for 3 minutes
- ➤ Set aside and let cool.
- ➤ Use a mixer, cream together the sugar and butter (if desired)
- ➤ Add the eggs one at a time until well-blended.
- ➤ Then the flour and toasted sesame seeds and mix until well-blended
- ➤ Drop spoonfuls of cookie dough onto a baking sheet
- ➤ Form them into round balls, about 1-inch in diameter, similar to a walnut.
- ➤ Put in the oven and bake for 5 to 7 minutes or until golden brown
- ➤ Let the cookies cool and enjoy.

NUTRITION INFORMATION: Calories: 218 fat: 12g protein: 4g carbs: 25g fiber: 2g sodium: 58mg

183 BUTTERY ALMOND COOKIES

Servings: 6   **Cook Time: 10 Min**   **Prep Time 5 Min**

INGREDIENTS:
- ✓ ½ cup sugar
- ✓ 8 tablespoons (1 stick) room temperature salted butter (optional)
- ✓ 1 large egg
- ✓ 1½ cups all-purpose flour
- ✓ cup ground almonds or almond flour

DIRECTIONS:

- ➤ Preheat the oven to 375°F (190°C).
- ➤ Use a mixer, cream together the sugar and butter (if desired).
- ➤ Add the egg and mix until combined.
- ➤ Alternately add the flour and ground almonds, ½ cup at a time, while the mixer is on slow.
- ➤ Once everything is combined, line a baking sheet with parchment paper
- ➤ Drop a tablespoon of dough on the baking sheet, keeping the cookies at least 2 inches apart.
- ➤ Put the baking sheet in the oven
- ➤ Bake just until the cookies start to turn brown around the edges, about 5 to 7 minutes

NUTRITION INFORMATION: Calories: 604 fat: 36g protein: 11g carbs: 63g fiber: 4g sodium: 181mg

184 HONEY WALNUT BAKLAVA

Servings: 8 **Cook Time: 1 H** **Prep Time 30 Min**

INGREDIENTS:
- ✓ 2 cups very finely chopped walnuts or pecans
- ✓ 1 teaspoon cinnamon
- ✓ 1 cup (2 sticks) unsalted butter, melted (optional)
- ✓ 1 (16-ounce / 454-g) package phyllo dough, thawed
- ✓ 1 (12-ounce / 340-g) jar honey

DIRECTIONS:
➢ Preheat the oven to 350°F (180°C).
➢ In a bowl, combine the chopped nuts and cinnamon.
➢ Use a brush, butter the sides and bottom of a 9-by-13-inch inch baking dish.
➢ Remove the phyllo dough from the package
➢ Cut it to the size of the baking dish using a sharp knife.
➢ Place one sheet of phyllo dough on the bottom of the dish
➢ Brush with butter, and repeat until you have 8 layers.
➢ Sprinkle ⅓ cup of the nut mixture over the phyllo layers
➢ Top with a sheet of phyllo dough, butter that sheet
➢ Repeat until you have 4 sheets of buttered phyllo dough.
➢ Sprinkle ⅓ cup of the nut mixture for another layer of nuts
➢ Repeat the layering of nuts and 4 sheets of buttered phyllo until all the nut mixture is gone
➢ The last layer should be 8 buttered sheets of phyllo.
➢ Before you bake, cut the baklava into desired shapes; traditionally this is diamonds, triangles, or squares.
➢ Bake the baklava for 1 hour or until the top layer is golden brown.
➢ While the baklava is baking, heat the honey in a pan just until it is warm and easy to pour.
➢ Once the baklava is done baking, immediately
➢ Pour the honey evenly over the baklava and let it absorb it, about 20 minutes
➢ Serve warm or at room temperature

NUTRITION INFORMATION: Calories: 754 fat: 46g protein: 8g carbs: 77g fiber: 3g sodium: 33mg

185 CREAMY RICE PUDDING

Servings: 6 **Cook Time: 45 Min** **Prep Time 5 Min**

INGREDIENTS:
- ✓ 1¼ cups long-grain rice
- ✓ 5 cups unsweetened almond milk
- ✓ 1 cup sugar
- ✓ 1 tablespoon rose water or orange blossom water
- ✓ 1 teaspoon cinnamon

DIRECTIONS:
➢ Rinse the rice under cold water for 30 seconds.
➢ Put the rice, milk, and sugar in a large pot
➢ Bring to a gentle boil while continually stirring.
➢ Turn the heat down to low and let simmer for 40 to 45 minutes
➢ Stir every 3 to 4 minutes so that the rice does not stick to the bottom of the pot.
➢ Add the rose water at the end and simmer for 5 minutes.
➢ Divide the pudding into 6 bowls
➢ Sprinkle the top with cinnamon
➢ Cool for at least 1 hour before serving. Store in the fridge.

NUTRITION INFORMATION: Calories: 323 fat: 7g protein: 9g carbs: 56g fiber: 1g sodium: 102mg

186 CREAM CHEESE AND RICOTTA CHEESECAKE

Servings: 10   **Cook Time: 1 H**   **Prep Time 5 Min**

INGREDIENTS:
- ✓ 2 (8-ounce / 227-g) packages full-fat cream cheese
- ✓ 1 (16-ounce / 454-g) container full-fat ricotta cheese
- ✓ 1½ cups granulated sugar
- ✓ 1 tablespoon lemon zest
- ✓ 5 large eggs
- ✓ Nonstick cooking spray

DIRECTIONS:
- ➤ Preheat the oven to 350°F (180°C).
- ➤ Use a mixer, blend together the cream cheese and ricotta cheese.
- ➤ Blend in the sugar and lemon zest.
- ➤ Blend in the eggs; drop in 1 egg at a time, blend for 10 seconds, and repeat.
- ➤ Line a 9-inch springform pan with parchment paper and nonstick spray
- ➤ Wrap the bottom of the pan with foil
- ➤ Pour the cheesecake batter into the pan.
- ➤ To make a water bath, get a baking or roasting pan larger than the cheesecake pan
- ➤ Fill the roasting pan about ⅓ of the way up with warm water
- ➤ Put the cheesecake pan into the water bath
- ➤ Place the whole thing in the oven
- ➤ Let the cheesecake bake for 1 hour.
- ➤ After baking is complete, remove the cheesecake pan from the water bath and remove the foil
- ➤ Let the cheesecake cool for 1 hour on the countertop
- ➤ Then put it in the fridge to cool for at least 3 hours before serving.

NUTRITION INFORMATION: Calories: 489 fat: 31g protein: 15g carbs: 42g fiber: 0g sodium: 264mg

187 VANILLA CAKE BITES

Makes 24 bites   **Cook Time: 45 Min**   **Prep Time 10 Min**

INGREDIENTS:
- ✓ 1 (12-ounce / 340-g) box butter cake mix
- ✓ ½ cup (1 stick) butter, melted (optional)
- ✓ 3 large eggs, divided
- ✓ 1 cup sugar
- ✓ 1 (8-ounce / 227-g) cream cheese
- ✓ 1 teaspoon vanilla extract

DIRECTIONS:
- ➤ Preheat the oven to 350°F (180°C).
- ➤ To make the first layer, in a medium bowl
- ➤ Blend the cake mix, butter (if desired), and 1 egg
- ➤ Then, pour the mixture into the prepared pan.
- ➤ In a separate bowl, to make layer 2, mix together sugar, cream cheese
- ➤ Add the remaining 2 eggs, and vanilla
- ➤ Pour this gently over the first layer
- ➤ Bake for 45 to 50 minutes and allow to cool.
- ➤ Cut the cake into 24 small squares.

NUTRITION INFORMATION: Calories: 160 fat: 8g protein: 2g carbs: 20g fiber: 0g sodium: 156mg

188 CRANBERRY ORANGE LOAF

Makes 1 loaf   **Cook Time: 45 Min**   **Prep Time 20 Min**

INGREDIENTS:

DOUGH:
- ✓ 3 cups all-purpose flour
- ✓ 1 (¼-ounce / 7-g) package quick-rise yeast
- ✓ ½ teaspoon salt
- ✓ ⅛ teaspoon ground cinnamon
- ✓ ⅛ teaspoon ground cardamom

- ✓ ½ cup water
- ✓ ½ cup almond milk
- ✓ ⅓ cup butter, cubed (optional)

CRANBERRY FILLING:
- ✓ 1 (12-ounce / 340-g) can cranberry sauce
- ✓ ½ cup chopped walnuts
- ✓ 2 tablespoons grated orange zest

- ✓ 2 tablespoons orange juice

DIRECTIONS:

- ➤ In a large bowl, combine the flour, yeast, salt, cinnamon, and cardamom.
- ➤ In a small pot, heat the water, almond milk, and butter (if desired) over medium-high heat
- ➤ Once it boils, reduce the heat to medium-low
- ➤ Simmer for 10 to 15 minutes, until the liquid thickens.

TO MAKE THE CRANBERRY FILLING:

- ➤ In a medium bowl, mix the cranberry sauce with walnuts
- ➤ Add orange zest, and orange juice in a large bowl.
- ➤ Assemble the bread
- ➤ Roll out the dough to about a 1-inch-thick and 10-by-7-inch-wide rectangle.
- ➤ Spread the cranberry filling evenly on the surface of the rolled-out dough

- ➤ Pour the liquid ingredients into the dry ingredients
- ➤ Use a wooden spoon or spatula
- ➤ Mix the dough until it forms a ball in the bowl.
- ➤ Put the dough in a greased bowl
- ➤ Cover tightly with a kitchen towel, and set aside for 1 hour.

- ➤ Leave a 1-inch border around the edges
- ➤ Starting with the long side, tuck the dough under with your fingertips and roll up the dough tightly
- ➤ Place the rolled-up dough in an "S" shape in a bread pan.
- ➤ Allow the bread to rise again, about 30 to 40 minutes.
- ➤ Preheat the oven to 350°F (180°C).
- ➤ Bake in a preheated oven, 45 minutes.

NUTRITION INFORMATION: Calories: 483 fat: 15g protein: 8g carbs: 79g fiber: 4g sodium: 232mg

189 APPLE PIE POCKETS

Servings: 6   **Cook Time: 15 Min**   **Prep Time 5 Min**

INGREDIENTS:

- ✓ 1 organic puff pastry, rolled out, at room temperature
- ✓ 1 Gala apple, peeled and sliced
- ✓ ¼ cup brown sugar
- ✓ ⅛ teaspoon ground cinnamon

- ✓ ⅛ teaspoon ground cardamom
- ✓ Nonstick cooking spray
- ✓ Honey, for topping

DIRECTIONS:

- ➤ Preheat the oven to 350°F (180°C).
- ➤ Cut the pastry dough into 4 even discs
- ➤ Peel and slice the apple
- ➤ In a small bowl, toss the slices with brown sugar, cinnamon, and cardamom.
- ➤ Spray a muffin tin very well with nonstick cooking spray
- ➤ Be sure to spray only the muffin holders you plan to use.

- ➤ Once sprayed, line the bottom of the muffin tin with the dough
- ➤ Place 1 or 2 broken apple slices on top
- ➤ Fold the remaining dough over the apple and drizzle with honey.
- ➤ Bake for 15 minutes or until brown and bubbly.

NUTRITION INFORMATION: Calories: 250 fat: 15g protein: 3g carbs: 30g fiber: 1g sodium: 98mg

190 BAKED PEARS WITH MASCARPONE CHEESE

Servings: 2   **Cook Time: 20 Min**   **Prep Time 10 Min**

INGREDIENTS:

- ✓ 2 ripe pears, peeled
- ✓ 1 tablespoon plus 2 teaspoons honey, divided
- ✓ 1 teaspoon vanilla, divided
- ✓ ¼ teaspoon ginger
- ✓ ¼ teaspoon ground coriander
- ✓ ¼ cup minced walnuts
- ✓ ¼ cup mascarpone cheese
- ✓ Pinch salt

DIRECTIONS:

- ➢ Preheat the oven to 350°F (180°C)
- ➢ Set the rack to the middle position. Grease a small baking dish.
- ➢ Cut the pears in half lengthwise
- ➢ Use a spoon, scoop out the core from each piece
- ➢ Place the pears with the cut side up in the baking dish.
- ➢ Combine 1 tablespoon of honey, ½ teaspoon of vanilla
- ➢ Add ginger, and coriander in a small bowl
- ➢ Pour this mixture evenly over the pear halves.
- ➢ Sprinkle walnuts over the pear halves.
- ➢ Bake for 20 minutes, or until the pears are golden and you're able to pierce them easily with a knife.
- ➢ While the pears are baking, mix the mascarpone cheese with the remaining 2 teaspoons honey, ½ teaspoon of vanilla, and a pinch of salt
- ➢ Stir well to combine.
- ➢ Divide the mascarpone among the warm pear halves and serve.

NUTRITION INFORMATION: Calories: 307 fat: 16g protein: 4g carbs: 43g fiber: 6g sodium: 89mg

191 ORANGE MUG CAKE

Servings: 2   **Cook Time: 2 Min**   **Prep Time 10 Min**

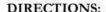

INGREDIENTS:

- ✓ 6 tablespoons flour
- ✓ 2 tablespoons sugar
- ✓ ½ teaspoon baking powder
- ✓ Pinch salt
- ✓ 1 teaspoon orange zest
- ✓ 1 egg
- ✓ 2 tablespoons olive oil
- ✓ 2 tablespoons freshly squeezed orange juice
- ✓ 2 tablespoons unsweetened almond milk
- ✓ ½ teaspoon orange extract
- ✓ ½ teaspoon vanilla extract

DIRECTIONS:

- ➢ In a small bowl, combine the flour, sugar, baking powder, salt, and orange zest.
- ➢ In a separate bowl, whisk together the egg, olive oil, orange juice, milk, orange extract, and vanilla extract.
- ➢ Pour the dry ingredients into the wet ingredients
- ➢ Stir to combine. The batter will be thick.
- ➢ Divide the mixture into two small mugs that hold at least 6 ounces / 170 g each, or 1 (12-ounce / 340-g) mug.
- ➢ Microwave each mug separately
- ➢ The small ones should take about 60 seconds, and one large mug should take about 90 seconds, but microwaves can vary
- ➢ The cake will be done when it pulls away from the sides of the mug.

NUTRITION INFORMATION: Calories: 302 fat: 17g protein: 6g carbs: 33g fiber: 1g sodium: 117mg

192 FRUIT AND NUT DARK CHOCOLATE BARK

Servings: 2   **Cook Time: 5 Min**   **Prep Time 15 Min**

INGREDIENTS:

- ✓ 2 tablespoons chopped nuts (almonds, pecans, walnuts, hazelnuts, pistachios, or any combination of those)

- ✓ 3 ounces (85 g) good-quality dark chocolate chips (about ⅔ cup)
- ✓ ¼ cup chopped dried fruit (apricots, blueberries, figs, prunes, or any combination of those)

DIRECTIONS:

- ➢ Line a sheet pan with parchment paper.
- ➢ Place the nuts in a skillet over medium-high
- ➢ Heat and toast them for 60 seconds, or just until they're fragrant.
- ➢ Place the chocolate in a microwave-safe glass bowl or measuring cup and microwave on high for 1 minute
- ➢ Stir the chocolate and allow any unmelted chips to warm and melt

- ➢ If necessary, heat for another 20 to 30 seconds, but keep a close eye on it to make sure it doesn't burn.
- ➢ Pour the chocolate onto the sheet pan
- ➢ Sprinkle the dried fruit and nuts over the chocolate evenly and gently pat in so they stick.
- ➢ Transfer the sheet pan to the refrigerator for at least 1 hour to let the chocolate harden.
- ➢ When solid, break into pieces
- ➢ Store any leftover chocolate in the refrigerator or freezer.

NUTRITION INFORMATION: Calories: 284 fat: 16g protein: 4g carbs: 39g fiber: 2g sodium: 2mg

193 GRILLED FRUIT SKEWERS

Servings: 2   **Cook Time: 10 Min**   **Prep Time 15 Min**

INGREDIENTS:

- ✓ ⅔ cup prepared labneh, or, if making your own, ⅔ cup full-fat plain Greek yogurt
- ✓ 2 tablespoons honey
- ✓ 1 teaspoon vanilla extract Pinch salt
- ✓ 3 cups fresh fruit cut into 2-inch chunks (pineapple, cantaloupe, nectarines, strawberries, plums, or mango)

DIRECTIONS:

- ➢ If making your own labneh, place a colander over a bowl and line it with cheesecloth
- ➢ Place the Greek yogurt in the cheesecloth and wrap it up
- ➢ Put the bowl in the refrigerator and let sit for at least 12 to 24 hours
- ➢ (Until it's thick like soft cheese)
- ➢ Mix honey, vanilla, and salt into labneh
- ➢ Stir well to combine and set it aside.

- ➢ Heat the grill to medium (about 300°F / 150°C) and oil the grill grate
- ➢ Alternatively, you can cook these on the stovetop in a heavy grill pan
- ➢ (cast iron works well).
- ➢ Thread the fruit onto skewers and grill for 4 minutes on each side
- ➢ (Or until fruit is softened and has grill marks on each side)
- ➢ Serve the fruit with labneh to dip.

NUTRITION INFORMATION: Calories: 292 fat: 6g protein: 5g carbs: 60g fiber: 4g sodium: 131mg

194 POMEGRANATE BLUEBERRY GRANITA

Servings: 2 **Cook Time: 10 Min** **Prep Time 15 Min**

INGREDIENTS:

- ✓ 1 cup frozen wild blueberries
- ✓ 1 cup pomegranate or pomegranate blueberry juice
- ✓ ¼ cup sugar
- ✓ ¼ cup water

DIRECTIONS:

- ➤ Combine the frozen blueberries and pomegranate juice in a saucepan and bring to a boil
- ➤ Reduce the heat and simmer for 5 minutes
- ➤ (Or until the blueberries start to break down)
- ➤ While the juice and berries are cooking
- ➤ Combine the sugar and water in a small microwave-safe bowl
- ➤ Microwave for 60 seconds, or until it comes to a rolling boil
- ➤ Stir to make sure all of the sugar is dissolved and set the syrup aside
- ➤ Combine the blueberry mixture and the sugar syrup in a blender
- ➤ Blend for 1 minute, or until the fruit is completely puréed.
- ➤ Pour the mixture into an 8-by-8-inch baking pan or a similar-sized bowl
- ➤ The liquid should come about ½ inch up the sides
- ➤ Let the mixture cool for 30 minutes, and then put it into the freezer.
- ➤ Every 30 minutes for the next 2 hours
- ➤ Scrape the granita with a fork to keep it from freezing solid.
- ➤ Serve it after 2 hours, or store it in a covered container in the freezer.

NUTRITION INFORMATION: Calories: 214 fat: 0g protein: 1g carbs: 54g fiber: 2g sodium: 15mg

195 CHOCOLATE DESSERT HUMMUS

Servings: 2 **Cook Time: 0 Min** **Prep Time 15 Min**

INGREDIENTS:

CARAMEL:

- ✓ 2 tablespoons coconut oil
- ✓ 1 tablespoon maple syrup

HUMMUS:

- ✓ ½ cup chickpeas, drained and rinsed
- ✓ 2 tablespoons unsweetened cocoa powder
- ✓ 1 tablespoon maple syrup, plus more to taste
- ✓ 1 tablespoon almond butter Pinch salt

- ✓ 2 tablespoons almond milk, or more as needed, to thin Pinch salt
- ✓ 2 tablespoons pecans

DIRECTIONS:

MAKE THE CARAMEL

- ➤ To make the caramel, put the coconut oil in a small microwave-safe bowl
- ➤ If it's solid, microwave it for about 15 seconds to melt it.

MAKE THE HUMMUS

- ➤ In a food processor, combine the chickpeas, cocoa powder
- ➤ Then maple syrup, almond milk, and pinch of salt, and process until smooth
- ➤ Scrape down the sides to make sure everything is incorporated.
- ➤ If the hummus seems too thick, add another tablespoon of almond milk.
- ➤ Stir in the maple syrup, almond butter, and salt.
- ➤ Place the caramel in the refrigerator for 5 to 10 minutes to thicken.

- ➤ Add the pecans and pulse 6 times to roughly chop them.
- ➤ Transfer the hummus to a serving bowl
- ➤ When the caramel is thickened, swirl it into the hummus
- ➤ Gently fold it in, but don't mix it in completely.
- ➤ Serve with fresh fruit or pretzels.

NUTRITION INFORMATION: Calories: 321 fat: 22g protein: 7g carbs: 30g fiber: 6g sodium: 100mg

196 BLACKBERRY LEMON PANNA COTTA

Servings: 2 **Cook Time: 10 Min** **Prep Time 20 Min**

INGREDIENTS:
- ✓ ¾ cup half-and-half, divided
- ✓ 1 teaspoon unflavored powdered gelatin
- ✓ ½ cup heavy cream
- ✓ 3 tablespoons sugar
- ✓ 1 teaspoon lemon zest
- ✓ 1 tablespoon freshly squeezed lemon juice
- ✓ 1 teaspoon lemon extract
- ✓ ½ cup fresh blackberries
- ✓ Lemon peels to garnish (optional)

DIRECTIONS:
- ➢ Place ¼ cup of half-and-half in a small bowl.
- ➢ Sprinkle the gelatin powder evenly over the half-and-half and set it aside for 10 minutes to hydrate.
- ➢ In a saucepan, combine the remaining ½ cup of half-
- ➢ Add-half, the heavy cream, sugar, lemon zest, lemon juice, and lemon extract
- ➢ Heat the mixture over medium heat for 4 minutes, or until it's barely simmering
- ➢ (Don't let it come to a full boil)
- ➢ Remove from the heat.
- ➢ When the gelatin is hydrated (it will look like applesauce)
- ➢ Add it into the warm cream mixture, whisking as the gelatin melts.
- ➢ If there are any remaining clumps of gelatin
- ➢ Strain the liquid or remove the lumps with a spoon.
- ➢ Pour the mixture into 2 dessert glasses or stemless wineglasses
- ➢ Refrigerate for at least 6 hours, or up to overnight.
- ➢ Serve with the fresh berries and garnish with some strips of fresh lemon peel, if desired.

NUTRITION INFORMATION: Calories: 422 fat: 33g protein: 6g carbs: 28g fiber: 2g sodium: 64mg

197 BERRY AND HONEY COMPOTE

Servings: 3 **Cook Time: 5 Min** **Prep Time 5 Min**

INGREDIENTS:
- ✓ ½ cup honey
- ✓ ¼ cup fresh berries
- ✓ 2 tablespoons grated orange zest

DIRECTIONS:
- ✓ 1.In a small saucepan, heat the honey, berries, and orange zest over medium-low heat for 2 to 5 minutes
- ✓ (Until the sauce thickens, or heat for 15 seconds in the microwave)
- ✓ Serve the compote drizzled over pancakes, muffins, or French toast.

NUTRITION INFORMATION: Calories: 272 fat: 0g protein: 1g carbs: 74g fiber: 1g sodium: 4mg

198 POMEGRANATE AND QUINOA DARK CHOCOLATE BARK

Servings: 6   **Cook Time: 13 Min**   **Prep Time 5 Min**

INGREDIENTS:

- ✓ Nonstick cooking spray
- ✓ ½ cup uncooked tricolor or regular quinoa
- ✓ ½ teaspoon kosher or sea salt
- ✓ 8 ounces (227 g) dark chocolate or 1 cup dark chocolate chips
- ✓ ½ cup fresh pomegranate seeds

DIRECTIONS:

- ➢ In a medium saucepan coated with nonstick cooking spray over medium heat
- ➢ Toast the uncooked quinoa for 2 to 3 minutes, stirring frequently
- ➢ Do not let the quinoa burn
- ➢ Remove the pan from the stove, and mix in the salt
- ➢ Set aside 2 tablespoons of the toasted quinoa to use for the topping.
- ➢ Break the chocolate into large pieces
- ➢ Put it in a gallon-size zip-top plastic bag
- ➢ Use a metal ladle or a meat pounder
- ➢ Pound the chocolate until broken into smaller pieces
- ➢ (If using chocolate chips, you can skip this step.)
- ➢ Dump the chocolate out of the bag into a medium, microwave
- ➢ (Safe bowl and heat for 1 minute on high in the microwave)
- ➢ Stir until the chocolate is completely melted
- ➢ Mix the toasted quinoa (except the topping you set aside) into the melted chocolate.
- ➢ Line a large, rimmed baking sheet with parchment paper
- ➢ Pour the chocolate mixture onto the sheet and spread it evenly
- ➢ (Until the entire pan is covered)
- ➢ Sprinkle the remaining 2 tablespoons of quinoa and the pomegranate seeds on top
- ➢ Use a spatula or the back of a spoon
- ➢ Press the quinoa and the pomegranate seeds into the chocolate.
- ➢ Freeze the mixture for 10 to 15 minutes, or until set
- ➢ Remove the bark from the freezer
- ➢ Break it into about 2-inch jagged pieces
- ➢ Store in a sealed container or zip-top plastic bag in the refrigerator until ready to serve.

NUTRITION INFORMATION: Calories: 268 fat: 11g protein: 4g carbs: 37g fiber: 2g sodium: 360mg

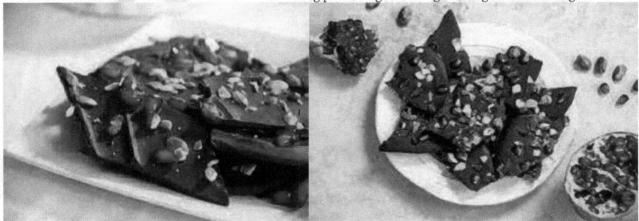

199 PECAN AND CARROT COCONUT CAKE

Servings: 12　　　　**Cook Time: 45 Min**　　　　**Prep Time 10 Min**

INGREDIENTS:

- ½ cup coconut oil, at room temperature, plus more for greasing the baking dish
- 2 teaspoons pure vanilla extract
- ¼ cup pure maple syrup 6 eggs
- ½ cup coconut flour
- 1 teaspoon baking powder 1 teaspoon baking soda
- ½ teaspoon ground nutmeg 1 teaspoon ground cinnamon
- ⅛ teaspoon sea salt
- ½ cup chopped pecans
- 3 cups finely grated carrots

DIRECTIONS:

- Preheat the oven to 350°F (180°C). Grease a 13-by-9-inch baking dish with coconut oil.
- Combine the vanilla extract, maple syrup, and ½ cup of coconut oil in a large bowl. Stir to mix well.
- Break the eggs in the bowl and whisk to combine well. Set aside.
- Combine the coconut flour, baking powder, baking soda, nutmeg, cinnamon, and salt in a separate bowl
- Stir to mix well.
- Make a well in the center of the flour mixture
- Then pour the egg mixture into the well
- Stir to combine well.
- Add the pecans and carrots to the bowl and toss to mix wel
- Pour the mixture in the single layer on the baking dish.
- Bake in the preheated oven for 45 minutes or until puffed and the cake spring back when lightly press with your fingers.
- Remove the cake from the oven
- Allow to cool for at least 15 minutes, then serve.

NUTRITION INFORMATION: Calories: 255 fat: 21g protein: 5g carbs: 12g fiber: 2g sodium: 202mg

200 AVOCADOS CHOCOLATE PUDDING

Servings: 4　　　　**Cook Time: 0 Min**　　　　**Prep Time 10 Min**

INGREDIENTS:

- 1 ripe avocados, halved and pitted
- ¼ cup unsweetened cocoa powder
- ¼ cup heavy whipping cream, plus more if needed
- 2 teaspoons vanilla extract
- 1 to 2 teaspoons liquid stevia or monk fruit extract (optional)
- ½ teaspoon ground cinnamon (optional)
- ¼ teaspoon salt
- Whipped cream, for serving (optional)

DIRECTIONS:

- Use a spoon, scoop out the ripe avocado into a blender or large bowl
- (If using an immersion blender)
- Mash well with a fork.
- Add the cocoa powder, heavy whipping cream, vanilla, sweetener (if using), cinnamon (if using), and salt
- Blend well until smooth and creamy, adding additional cream, 1 tablespoon at a time, if the mixture is too thick.
- Cover and refrigerate for at least 1 hour before serving
- Serve chilled with additional whipped cream, if desired.

NUTRITION INFORMATION: Calories: 230 fat: 21g protein: 3g carbs: 10g fiber: 5g sodium: 163mg

INTRODUCTION

GLUTEN-FREE DIET

More than 20 million people around the world have adopted a gluten-free diet and radically changed the way they eat. Healthy eating advocates strongly claim that eliminating wheat and other gluten-enriched products from their diets has helped them achieve healthier bodies, clearer minds and happier souls. We learn about the science behind this controversial protein and how it affects the balance of the human body:

THE COMPOSITION OF GLUTEN

In its simplest form, gluten is a protein found in food products made from wheat, barley, rye and other grains. It is composed of two proteins: glutenin and gliadin. The reason why gluten grains are used in food preparation is their chemical composition, which gives elasticity to the food, making it softer and easier to chew. Bread has been shown to contain more gluten than most foods because more gluten fibres are extracted during the kneading process and bind with other proteins. However, processed foods and artificial flavour enhancers have been found to contain gluten, as well as other chemicals that are harmful to the body.

HOW IS GLUTEN HARMFUL TO THE BODY?

High consumption of foods enriched with gluten triggers a negative autoimmune response. In the body, making it more prone to allergies, illnesses and disorders. This reaction can be attributed to the body's reaction to gliadin, a subprotein of gluten that creates abnormal activity in the digestive tract. Once gluten enters the body and adheres to the wall of the digestive tract, the immune system considers it a harmful element that must be eliminated. The immune system automatically attacks gluten, damaging healthy stomach cells in the process. The damaged cells in the gut become a passageway for bacteria and other harmful chemicals to enter the body. Diseases that are associated with regular gluten intake include celiac disease, irritable bowel syndrome, leaky gut syndrome, anaemia, fatigue, food allergies and brain damage. Although coeliac disease is known to be genetically inherited, other diseases have arisen as a result of gluten intolerance caused by eating huge portions of cereal products.

BENEFITS OF A GLUTEN-FREE DIET

People who have taken a turn for the better and eliminated gluten from their diet have experienced the wonders of clean, healthy eating. Removing wheat products from the diet and replacing them with fruits, vegetables, dairy products and lean meats helps cleanse the body and protect cells from degeneration. Here are some of the health benefits of a gluten-free diet: easier weight control fewer cravings for unhealthy foods food allergies are eliminated treating coeliac disease and other autoimmune diseases by reducing IBS symptoms lower risk of stomach problems lower cholesterol and blood sugar levels reduced risk of heart disease and cancer more energy for weight loss activities happier mood easier management of symptoms of brain disorders in people with autism, epilepsy and schizophrenia

GLUTEN-FREE FOOD CHECKLIST

Before you embark on your journey to a healthier gluten-free lifestyle, it's important to know which foods should be on your shopping list and which should be eliminated from your pantry. Here's a list of foods that will help you prepare healthier meals:

SAFE GLUTEN-FREE FOODS

Gluten-free flours and cereals such as almond flour, millet, amaranth, buckwheat, sorghum, maize flour, potato flour, quinoa, rice (brown, white), teff flour, gluten-free oats. Fresh fruit, vegetables and herbs Beans, pulses and soybeans Nuts and healthy seeds Canned fruit, vegetables and fruit juices, as long as they do not contain artificial sweeteners or additives. Dairy products such as butter, milk, eggs, cream, real cheese, gluten-free yoghurt Red meat, chicken and seafood unless breaded or dipped in gluten-enriched marinades. Healthy oils, e.g. olive, coconut, sesame, canola Sweeteners, e.g. sugar, honey, maple syrup, coconut sugar, agave. Spices and condiments, e.g. vinegar, gluten-free soy sauce, coconut aminos, ground spices, dried herbs.Alcoholic drinks. Baked goods such as pectin powder, xantham and guar gum, tapioca, baking powder, baking soda, vanilla.

GLUTEN PRODUCTS TO AVOID

Recipes enriched with wheat flour, couscous, semolina, kamut, spelt, durum wheat, triticale, modified wheat starch, cake flour.

Malt products such as malt vinegar, malt syrup, malt flavouring Barley products such as liquorice, imitation seafood, beer Artificial seasonings, sauces and marinades Rye processed cheese and spreadable cheese. Bread and baked goods such as cakes, doughnuts, muffins, pretzels. To create a healthier cuisine, always check the grocery shop for gluten-free alternatives to your favourite foods. Otherwise, it's always best to stick to using organic and wheat-free ingredients when preparing meals for you and the whole family. Switching to a gluten-free lifestyle may seem challenging at first, but its benefits are worth any simple changes you're willing to make in your daily eating habits. Eating healthy and gluten-free will help you achieve overall well-being and a better life ahead of you. Gluten-free meals can be prepared in various ways: grilled, pan-fried, baked or steamed. However, an easier way to prepare these delicious recipes is to use a slow cooker. This way, you get the same flavour and nutritional value without having to spend countless hours in the kitchen.The following section will discuss the advantages of a slow cooker.Your gluten-free cooking and some tips on how it can help beginner cooks prepare nutritious and delicious meals

Author's note: This book has given you all the information you need to do this diet correctly and do it right. It is essential to understand what you are getting into when you embark on this diet, and this book gave you valuable information that you can use to your advantage and avoid the problems that can come with this diet. You want to stay healthy and make sure that your body can do what it needs to do. As with anything, we emphasize that if something seems wrong or unnatural, you will need to see a doctor to make sure you are safe and that your body can handle this diet. Use the knowledge in this book to get amazing recipes and learn directions for excellent meals for yourself. Consult your doctor before to starting new diet.

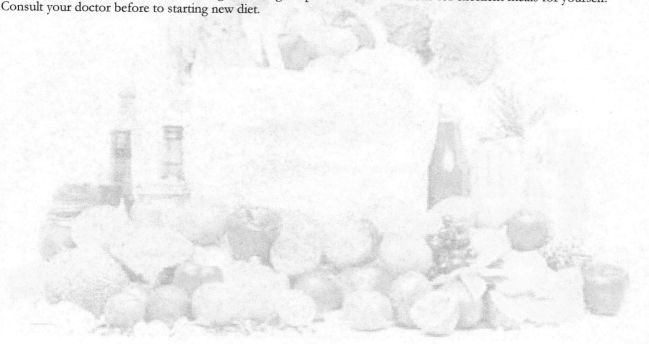

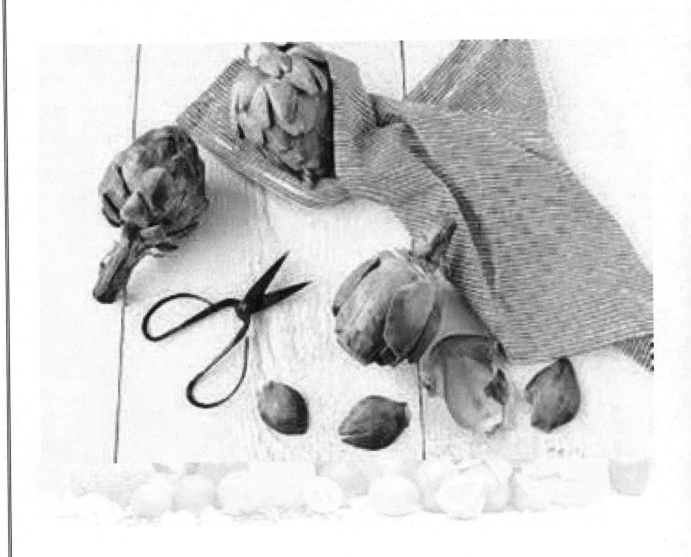

1. TURKEY AND ARTICHOKES BREAKFAST CASSEROLE

Preparation Time: 15 minutes   **Cooking Time:** 60 minutes   **Servings:** 12

Ingredients:

- 1 1/2 pound ground turkey 2 green onion, sliced
- 1 medium green bell pepper, diced 14 ounces artichoke hearts, chopped 2 ½ cups fresh baby spinach
- 1/2 of a medium onion, peeled, diced 1/2 teaspoon cumin
- ¾ teaspoon ground black pepper 1/2 teaspoon oregano
- 1 teaspoon salt
- 1 teaspoon red chili powder 2 tablespoons avocado oil 16 eggs, beaten

Directions:

- Switch on the oven, then set it to 375 degrees F and let preheat.
- Meanwhile, take a skillet pan, place it over medium heat, add oil and when hot, add onion and green bell pepper.
- Then add turkey, season with cumin, black pepper, oregano, salt, and red chili powder, stir well and cook for 10 minutes until meat is thoroughly cooked and nicely browned.
- Add 2 cups spinach into cooked meat, stir well and continue cooking for 2 minutes until spinach leaves have wilted.
- Take a 9 by 13 inches casserole dish or twelve oven safe meal prep glass containers, spoon in the turkey-spinach mixture, spread it evenly, and then top with artichokes.
- Beat the eggs, pour it over artichokes in the casserole
- Sprinkle with green onion and remaining spinach and bake the casserole for 45 minutes until thoroughly cooked.
- For meal prepping, let casserole or containers cool completely
- Then cover the casserole well with aluminum foil or close the containers with lid and store in the refrigerator for up to five days or freeze for three months.
- Reheat casserole in the microwave until hot and serve

2. GRANOLA

Preparation Time 15 minutes   **Cooking Time:** 20 minutes   **Servings:** 10

Ingredients:

- 1 cup raisins
- 3 cups rolled oats, old-fashioned 1 cup sliced almonds
- 1/2 teaspoon ground cinnamon 1/2 teaspoon salt
- 1/2 cup honey 1/2 cup olive oil

Directions:

- Switch on the oven, then set it to 300 degrees F, then place the baking rack in the middle of the oven and let preheat.
- Place oil in a large bowl, whisk in cinnamon, salt, and honey until combined, then add almonds and oats and stir until well coated.
- Take a rimmed baking sheet, line it with parchment paper, spoon oats mixture on it
- Then spread it in an even layer and bake for 20 minutes until granola is golden brown, stirring halfway through.
- Sprinkle raisins on top of granola, press it lightly and then let the granola cool.
- Break granola into small pieces, then transfer granola into an airtight container
- Store for up to one month at room temperature.
- When ready to eat, add some of the granola in a bowl, pour in milk, top with berries and serve

3. ALMOND CRANBERRY CHOCOLATE GRANOLA BARS

Preparation Time 20 minutes   **Cooking Time: 25** minutes   **Servings:12**

Ingredients:
- 1 1/2 cups rolled oats, old-fashioned
- 1/4 cup chocolate chips
- 3/4 cup sliced almonds
- 1/3 cup cranberries, dried
- 1/3 cup honey

- 1/8 teaspoon salt
- 2 tablespoons brown sugar
- 3 tablespoons butter, unsalted
- 1/2 teaspoon vanilla extract, unsweetened
- 2 tablespoons peanut butter

Directions:
- Switch on the oven, then set it to 325 degrees and let preheat.
- Take a medium saucepan, place it over medium-low heat
- Add the butters, honey, sugar, salt, and vanilla
- Stir well until combined and cook for 5 minutes until the sugar has dissolved and butter has melted.
- Meanwhile, place oats in a medium bowl, add almonds and stir until mixed.
- Pour in prepared honey mixture, stir until well combined, and let the mixture stand at room temperature for 10 minutes.

Then add chocolate chips and cranberries and fold until just mixed.

Take a 9 by 9 inches casserole dish, line it with parchment sheet, spoon in prepared oats mixture

Spread and firmly press into the pan by using the back of a glass and bake for 25 minutes until crunchy.

Let the granola cool in the pan on a wire rack, then cut into twelve bars

Store in an airtight container for up to one week at room temperature or refrigerate for up to one month.

4. CINNAMON RAISIN GRANOLA

Preparation Time: 10 minutes   **Cooking Time:30** minutes   **Servings:5**

Ingredients:
- 1 cup shredded coconut, unsweetened
- 1/2 cup raisins
- 1 cup pumpkin seeds
- 1/2 cup chopped pecans
- 1 cup sunflower seeds
- 1/2 cup sliced almonds

- 1/4 teaspoon salt
- 1/2 teaspoon allspice
- 1 tablespoon cinnamon
- 1 teaspoon vanilla extract, unsweetened
- 2 tablespoons maple syrup
- 1/3 cup coconut oil
- 1/4 cup honey

Directions:
- Switch on the oven, then set it to 300 degrees F and let it preheat.
- Meanwhile, place all the ingredients in a large bowl, except for vanilla, maple syrup, oil, and honey and stir until well mixed.
- Take a saucepan, place it over low heat, add vanilla, maple syrup, oil, and honey, stir well and cook for 5 minutes until melted.
- Meanwhile, take a 10 by 15 inches baking sheet and then line it with parchment paper.

- Pour this mixture over granola mixture in the bowl and mix by hand until combined.
- Transfer granola mixture onto the prepared baking sheet
- Spread it evenly, and bake for 25 minutes until golden brown, stirring halfway through.
- Cool the granola on a wire rack and then break it into small pieces.
- Transfer granola into an airtight container and then store for up to one month at room temperature.
- When ready to eat, add some of the granola in a bowl, pour in milk, top with berries and serve

5. AVOCADO BREAKFAST BOWL

Preparation Time: 10 minutes   **Cooking Time:**30 minutes   Servings:2

Ingredients:
- Water (.5 cup)
- Red quinoa (.25 cup)
- Olive oil (1.5 tsp.)
- Eggs (2)

- Black pepper & salt (1 pinch/as desired)
- Seasoned salt (.25 tsp.)
- Avocado (1 diced)
- Crumbled feta cheese (2 tbsp.)

Directions:

Toss the quinoa, salt, and water into a rice cooker. Set the timer for 15 minutes.

Warm oil in a skillet using the medium temperature setting. Cook the eggs, pepper, and seasoned salt.

- ix the eggs and quinoa. Top them off with a portion of the feta and avocado

6. BABY SPINACH OMELET

Preparation Time: 10 minutes   **Cooking Time:**30 minutes   Servings:2

Ingredients:
- Eggs (2)
- Baby spinach leaves (1 cup)
- Onion powder (.25 tsp.)

- Grated parmesan cheese (1 tbsp. + .5 tsp.)
- Ground nutmeg (⅛ tsp.)
- Black pepper & salt (to your liking)

Directions:
- Whisk the eggs and stir in the spinach, parmesan, pepper, salt, nutmeg, and onion powder.
- Prepare a skillet using a cooking oil spray. Cook them for about three minutes, until partially cooked.

- Flip them over with a spatula and continue cooking for another two to three minutes.
- Lower the heat and simmer on low until it is done (2-3 min.). Serve immediately

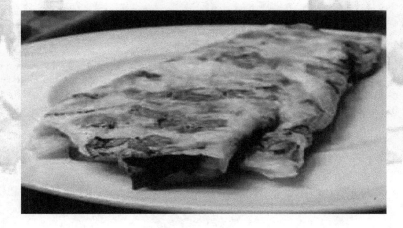

7. BACON CHEDDAR DROP BISCUITS

Preparation Time: 10 minutes   **Cooking Time:** 20 minutes   **Servings:** 10

Ingredients:
- Almond flour (1.5 cups)
- Onion powder (1 tsp.)
- Baking powder (1 tbsp.)
- Garlic salt (1 tsp.)
- Baking soda (.5 tsp.)
- Dried parsley (1 tbsp.)
- Bacon (4 slices)
- Eggs (2)
- Sour cream (.5 cup)
- Bacon grease melted (1 tbsp.)
- Shredded cheddar cheese (1/3 cup)
- Shredded smoky bacon cheddar cheese (1/3 cup)
- Melted grass-fed butter (3 tbsp.)
- Swerve confectioners or powdered erythritol (.5 tsp.)

Directions:
- Set the oven temperature in advance to 425° Fahrenheit.
- Prepare a baking tin with a layer of baking paper.
- Cook and crumble the bacon.
- Add the baking powder, flour, onion powder, baking soda, and garlic salt into a mixing container using a fork or whisk.
- Combine the eggs in with the melted butter, bacon grease, bacon, parsley, sour cream.
- Fold the cheese and combine everything.
- Scoop the biscuit mixture onto the prepared pan.
- Bake them for 11 to 15 minutes

8. BANANA COCONUT BAKED OATMEAL

Preparation Time: 10 minutes   **Cooking Time:** 20 minutes   **Servings:** 2

Ingredients:
- Ground flaxseed (1 tbsp.)
- Water (3 tbsp.)
- Gluten-free rolled oats (1 cup)
- Unsweetened shredded coconut (2 tbsp.)
- Ground cinnamon (.25 tsp.)
- Nutmeg (1/8 tsp.)
- Baking powder (.25 tsp.)
- Coconut milk beverage from the carton, not the can (1 cup)
- Mashed ripe banana (.33 cup/about 1 medium)
- Pure vanilla extract (.25 tsp.)
- Also Needed: Ramekins (3)

Directions:
- Warm the oven to reach 350° Fahrenheit. Spritz the ramekins with a cooking oil spray.
- Whisk the flaxseed meal and three tablespoons of warm water. Wait for about five minutes.
- Combine the shredded coconut, oats, nutmeg, cinnamon, and baking powder.
- Whisk the coconut milk, vanilla extract, and mashed banana into the bowl with the flaxseed mixture.
- Pour the dry fixings into the wet and stir until incorporated. Fill the ramekins and garnish with banana slices.
- Bake until the oatmeal is puffed and set (20 min.) to serve right away

9. BROCCOLI AND RED PEPPER EGG MUFFINS

Preparation Time: 10 minutes   **Cooking Time:** 20 minutes   Servings: 8

Ingredients:
- 1/2 cup roasted red pepper, cored, diced
- 1/2 cup broccoli florets, riced
- 1/2 teaspoon ground black pepper
- 1/2 teaspoon salt
- 1/2 teaspoon garlic powder
- 1 tablespoon coconut milk, unsweetened
- 4 eggs
- 4 egg whites

Directions:
- Switch on the oven, then set it to 325 degrees F, and let it preheat.
- Meanwhile, whisk the eggs and egg whites in a large bowl
- Then beat in black pepper, salt, garlic powder, and milk until combined.
- Then add red pepper and riced broccoli and stir until mixed.
- Take an eight cups muffin pan, grease its cups with oil, then evenly fill with prepared broccoli and red pepper mixtur
- Bake for 20 minutes until eggs are set and muffins are firm in the center.
- When done, take out muffins from the muffin pan and let cool on the wire rack.
- For meal prep, wrap each muffin with aluminum foil and refrigerate for up to five days or freeze for up to one month.
- When ready to eat, reheat the muffin in the microwave until hot and serve

10. PANCAKES

Preparation Time: **10** minutes   **Cooking Time:** **12** minutes   Servings: 4

Ingredients:
- 1 cup coconut flour
- 1/4 cup coconut oil, melted
- 1 1/2 cups almond milk, unsweetened
- 8 eggs
- Strawberries, fresh, for topping

Directions:
- Place flour in a large bowl, add oil, milk, and eggs and beat until smooth batter comes together.
- Take a skillet pan, place it over medium heat, grease it with oil and when hot
- Add 3 tablespoons of batter per pancake in it and cook the pancake for 3 minutes per side until nicely golden from both sides.
- Cook more pancakes in the same manner until all the batter is used up.
- Let pancakes cool, then divide them evenly between four ovenproof meal prep containers
- Stack pancakes with wax paper in between, and add strawberries.
- Cover the containers with lid and freeze for up to two months.
- When ready to eat, reheat pancakes in the microwave for 2 minutes until hot and serve

11. BREAKFAST POWER BOWL

Preparation Time: 10 minutes   **Cooking Time:**0 minutes   **Servings:**2

Ingredients:
- 1 cup shredded carrots
- 1/2 cup lentils, cooked
- 2 cups quinoa, cooked
- 1 medium avocado, peeled, pitted, thinly sliced
- 1 cup shredded red cabbage
- 1/2 teaspoon garlic powder
- 1/4 teaspoon cumin
- 6 eggs, hard-boiled

Directions:
- Place cooked quinoa in a large bowl, add lentils, sprinkle with cumin and garlic powder and stir until combined.
- Take meal prep containers, fill them evenly with quinoa mixture, and then evenly add shredded carrots and cabbage.
- Peel the boiled eggs, then cut each egg in half and place them on top with quinoa along with avocado slices.
- Cover the containers with lid and store in the refrigerator for up to five days and serve when required

12. SAUSAGE-HASH BROWN CASSEROLE

Preparation Time: 45 minutes   **Cooking Time:**45 minutes   **Servings:**6

Ingredients:
- 6 sausages, sliced
- 1 cup fresh spinach
- 4 cups shredded potatoes
- ½ teaspoon ground black pepper
- 2/3 teaspoon salt
- 1 1/3 cup egg whites 6 eggs

Directions:
- Switch on the oven, then set it to 350 degrees F and let preheat.
- Meanwhile, take a skillet pan, place it over medium heat, grease it with oil and when hot, add sausage
- Cook for 3 minutes per side until sauté.
- Place eggs and egg whites in a bowl, whisk until blended, then add sausage, spinach, and potatoes and mix well until combined.
- Take a 9 by 13 inches casserole dish or six heatproof meal prep glass containers, spoon in sausage mixture, and bake the casserole for 45 minutes until thoroughly cooked.
- For meal prepping, let casserole or containers cool completely
- Then cover the casserole well with aluminum foil or close the containers with lid
- Store in the refrigerator for up to five days or freeze for three months.
- Reheat casserole in the microwave until hot and serve

13. OMELET MUFFINS

Preparation Time: 10 minutes   **Cooking Time:40** minutes   Servings:6

Ingredients:

- 4 scallions, sliced
- 2 cups chopped broccoli
- 3 slices of bacon, chopped
- ½ teaspoon ground black pepper

- ½ teaspoon salt
- 8 eggs
- ½ cup milk
- 1 cup shredded cheddar cheese

Directions:

- Switch on the oven, then set it to 325 degrees F and let it preheat.
- Meanwhile, take a skillet pan, place it over medium heat and when hot, add bacon and cook for 5 minutes until cooked and crispy.
- Transfer cooked bacon to a plate lined with paper towels and set aside until required.
- Add scallion and broccoli into the pan, stir well and cook for 5 minutes until softened, set aside and let cool for 5 minutes.

- In the meantime, place cheese in a bowl, add eggs, pour in milk, season with black pepper and salt, and whisk until combined.
- Then add bacon and broccoli and stir until well mixed.
- Take a twelve cups muffin pan, grease its cups with oil, then fill the cups evenly with broccoli mixture
- Bake for 30 minutes until firm.
- When done, take out muffins from the pan and let them cool on a wire rack.
- For meal prep, wrap each muffin with aluminum foil and refrigerate for up to five days or freeze for up to one month.
- When ready to eat, reheat the muffin in the microwave until hot and serve

14. PARSNIP HASH BROWNS

Preparation Time: 10 minutes   **Cooking Time:10** minutes   Servings:6

Ingredients:

- 16 ounces waxy potato
- 12 ounces parsnip
- 1 small white onion, halved and sliced

- ½ tablespoon minced garlic
- 1 egg, beaten
- 4 tablespoons olive oil

Directions:

- Peel the potatoes and parsnip, grate them by using a food processor, then wrap potatoes and parsnip in a kitchen cloth
- Squeeze out moisture as much as possible.
- Place squeeze potatoes and parsnip in a bowl, add egg, garlic, and onion and whisk until well combined.
- Shape the mixture into six flat cakes, then place them on a cookie sheet lined with parchment paper and freeze until hard.

- For meal prep, transfer frozen the hash browns in a plastic bag and freeze in the freezer for up to three months.
- When ready to eat, place a skillet over medium heat
- Add oil and hash brown and cook for 15 minutes until hot and nicely browned on both sides, flipping every 5 minutes.
- Serve hash browns with cherry tomatoes and poached eggs

15. CHORIZO BREAKFAST SKILLET

Preparation Time: 10 minutes   **Cooking Time: 20** minutes   **Servings:2**

Ingredients:
- Olive oil (2 tsp.)
- Small onion (1)
- Chorizo cold cuts (6 slices)
- Cherry tomatoes (.5 cup)
- Sun-dried tomatoes (3)
- Eggs (4)
- Fresh basil (1 handful - slivered)

Directions:
- Quarter the cold cuts and cut the cherry tomatoes into halves.
- Warm oil in a skillet using the medium temperature setting.
- Cut the onion in half and slice it. Toss it in the pan to sauté for about two minutes.
- Mix in the chorizo, in a single layer, and cook it for two to three minutes.
- Add the cherry tomatoes with the cut side down. Sauté them for two to three minutes.
- Chop and fold in the sun-dried tomatoes and combine all of the fixings together
- Use a spoon to make four mini craters in the four corners of the pan and crack four eggs (one into each hole)
- Sprinkle with the pepper and salt.
- Continue cooking until the eggs are set. Serve with fresh basil

16. GF FRENCH TOAST WITH BACON-INFUSED SYRUP

Preparation Time: 5 minutes   **Cooking Time:10** minutes   **Servings:4**

Ingredients:
- Gluten-free bread (8 slices)
- Large eggs (3)
- Milk or dairy substitute (.5 cup)
- Vanilla (1.25 tsp.)
- Dark brown sugar (.25 cup)
- GF cornstarch (2 tbsp.)
- GF baking powder (1 tsp.)
- Salt (big pinch)
- Canola oil (1 tbsp.)
- Unsalted butter (2 tbsp.)
- The Syrup:
- Bacon (2 slices)
- Water (.33 cup)
- Granulated sugar (.5 cup)
- Salt (1 pinch)
- Packed dark brown sugar (.5 cup)
- Vanilla (1.5 tsp.)

Directions:
- Warm the oven at 350° Fahrenheit
- Place eight slices of bread on a rack and bake them for approximately five minutes
- Remove it and let it cool.
- Cook the bacon until it is crispy. Cool and crumble for later.
- In a flat dish, whisk the eggs, milk, vanilla, dark brown sugar, cornstarch, baking powder, and salt to remove all lumps.
- Warm the oil and butter in a frying pan using the med-high temperature setting.
- Dip the sliced bread into the batter, flipping once. Carefully transfer them to the frying pan
- Cook them for three to five minutes on each side. Lower the burner setting as needed.
- Make the Syrup: Add one slice of crumbled bacon and the rest of the fixings in a large microwave-safe bowl
- Reserve the second slice of bacon for the garnish. Whisk the syrup thoroughly.
- Microwave the syrup on high for 45 seconds. Stir well. Return the dish to the microwave for 60 seconds
- Stir and serve the toast warm with the bacon-infused syrup

17. HASH & SPINACH EGGS

Preparation Time: 10 minutes   **Cooking Time:** 30 minutes   **Servings: 4**

Ingredients:
- Russet potatoes (3 medium)
- Olive oil (2 tbsp.)
- Small onion (1)
- Fresh spinach (1 cup)
- Garlic powder (.5 tsp.)
- Large eggs (4)
- Freshly cracked black pepper & salt (.25 tsp. each)

Directions:
- Thoroughly scrub the potatoes and dot them using a fork. Pop them into the microwave for eight minutes or so until they're tender.
- Roughly chop the potatoes (.5-inch bits) and toss them into a skillet with oil using the med-high temperature setting.
- Chop the spinach and onion, and mince the garlic. Sauté them for about five to six minutes.
- Press the spinach and hash into the pan. Make four "wells" in the center and add an egg to each one
- Sprinkle them with the pepper and salt.
- Place a lid on the pan and cook for about ten minutes until it's as desired and serve

18. RASPBERRY-PEACH CRISP OVERNIGHT OATS

Preparation Time: 5 minutes   **Cooking Time:** 5 minutes   **Servings: 2**

Ingredients:
- Vanilla Greek yogurt (12 oz.)
- GF raw old-fashioned oats (2/3 cup)
- Milk - any type (.25 cup)
- Optional: Chia seeds (2 tsp.)
- Vanilla (1 tsp.)
- Chopped peaches (2)
- Raspberries (6 oz.)
- Sliced almonds (.25 cup)

Directions:
- In a large mixing container, combine the vanilla, chia seeds, milk, yogurt, and oats.
- Scoop a fourth of the mixture into the jars with the peaches, berries, and one tablespoon of the almonds.
- Repeat the layer and close the lids.
- You can store them in the fridge for two to three days

19. DELICIOUS BAGELS

Preparation Time: 5 minutes   **Cooking Time:** 20 minutes   **Servings: 6**

Ingredients:
- Melted butter (1/3 cup)
- Eggs (6)
- Cinnamon (1 tbsp.)
- Sugar-free vanilla extract (2 tsp.)
- Stevia glycerite (5-10 drops) or Swerve sweetener (1 to 1.5 tbsp.)
- Maple extract (1 tsp.)
- Salt (.5 tsp.)
- Sifted coconut flour (.5 cup)
- Xanthan gum or guar gum (.5 tsp. or optional)
- Baking powder (.5 tsp.)

Directions:
- Set the oven temperature at 400° Fahrenheit. Lightly grease a donut pan.
- Blend the eggs with the cinnamon, vanilla extract, maple extract, stevia, salt, and butter.
- Whisk the coconut flour with the baking powder and guar/xanthan gum.
- Combine everything and spoon it into the pan. Bake the bagels for 15 minutes

20. GARLIC COCONUT FLOUR BAGELS

Preparation Time: 5minutes   **Cooking Time:** 30 minutes   Servings:6

Ingredients:
- Melted butter (1/3 cup)
- Sifted coconut flour (.5 cup)
- Optional: Guar gum or xanthan gum (2 tsp.)

- Eggs (6)
- Salt (.5 tsp.)
- Garlic powder (1.5 tsp.)
- Baking powder (.5 tsp.)

Directions:
- Set the oven at 400° Fahrenheit.
- Lightly grease a donut pan.
- Blend the eggs, butter, salt, and garlic powder.
- Transfer the bagels from the pan to cool or serve

- Combine coconut flour with baking powder and guar or xanthan gum.
- Whisk the coconut flour mixture into the batter until there are no lumps.
- Scoop it into the pan. Set a timer to bake for 15 minutes.
- Wait for it to cool on a wire rack for 10-15 minutes

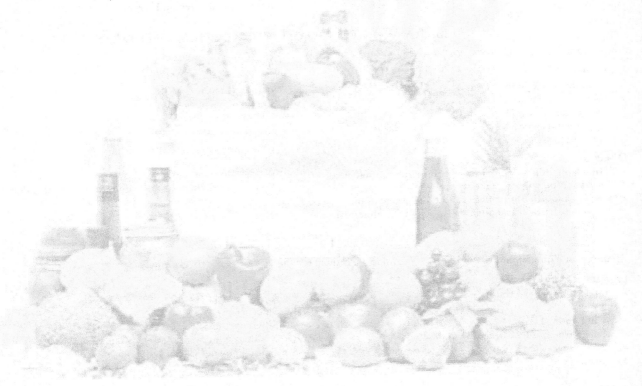

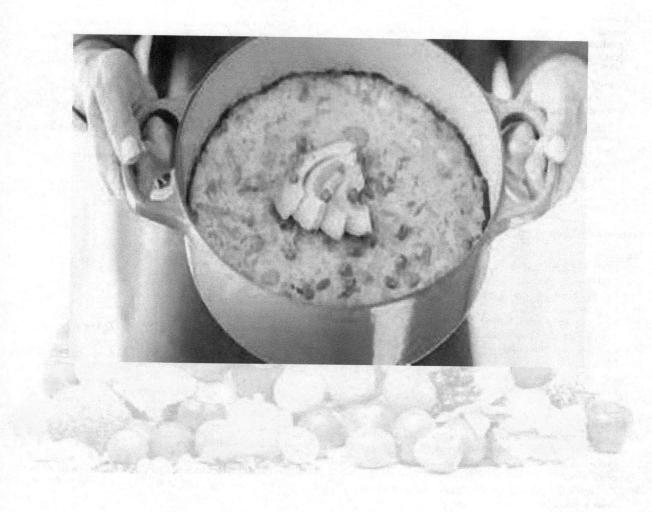

21. BUFFALO CHICKEN CASSEROLE

Preparation Time: 10 minutes   **Cooking Time:** 55 minutes   **Servings:** 4

Ingredients:
- 1/2 cup diced carrots
- 15 ounces cauliflower florets, riced
- 1 small white onion, peeled, diced
- ½ teaspoon minced garlic
- 1 pound chicken breast, skinless, cooked, shredded
- 1/4 teaspoon ground black pepper
- 2 tablespoons olive oil
- 1/2 cup egg whites
- 3/4 cup buffalo sauce

Directions:
- Switch on the oven, then set it to 400 degrees F and let it preheat.
- Take a skillet pan, place it over medium heat
- Add oil and when hot, add onion, celery, and carrots and cook for 5 minutes or until softened.
- Then transfer vegetables to a bowl, add remaining ingredients and mix well until combined.
- Take a baking pan or casserole dish, line it with parchment sheet, spoon in the prepared mixture
- Then cover with aluminum foil and bake for 25 minutes.
- Uncover the pan and continue baking for 25 minutes until casserole has set and the top is nicely golden brown.
- When the casserole has cooked, remove it from the oven and let it cool completely.
- Then divide the casserole into four pieces and place each casserole piece in a heatproof glass meal prep container.
- Cover meal prep containers with lid and freeze for up to two months.
- When ready to eat, reheat the casserole in the microwave until hot
- Cover the top if it gets too brown, and then serve with a green salad

22. CHICKEN MASON JAR SALAD

Preparation Time: 10 minutes   **Cooking Time:** 0 minutes   **Servings:** 4

Ingredients:
FOR THE SALAD:
- 2 tablespoons sliced green onions
- 2 cups sliced napa cabbage
- 1 cup grated carrots
- 1 1/3 cup snap peas, halved
- 2 cups shredded rotisserie chicken
- 1 red pepper, julienned
- 1 1/3 cups cucumber, sliced
- 2 cups baby spinach, sliced
- 1 cup cashews, unsalted

FOR THE SESAME DRESSING:
- 1 tablespoon minced ginger 2 tablespoons diced cilantro 3 tablespoons soy sauce
- 1 tablespoon honey
- tablespoon olive oil
- ½ teaspoon minced garlic
- tablespoons apple cider vinegar 2 1/2 tablespoons sesame oil
- 1 teaspoon sriracha sauce 1 teaspoon sesame seeds

Directions:
- Prepare the dressing and for this, place all its ingredients in a bowl and whisk until combined.
- Place cabbage in a bowl, add spinach and toss until combined.
- Assemble the salad jar and for this, take four 64-ounce mason salad jar
- Work on one mason jar at a time, spoon 3 tablespoons of prepared salad dressing into a salad jar, then 1/3 cup snap peas and top with ¼ cup shredded carrots.
- Add 1/3 cup cucumber, top with 1 cup of cabbage mixture, ½ cupchicken, then add ¼ cup cashews and sprinkle with green onions.
- Prepare remaining salad jars in the same manner, cover with the lid, and store in the freezer for up to four days.
- Serve straight away

23. QUICK GLUTEN-FREE SEAFOOD SOUP

Preparation Time: 10 minutes   **Cooking Time**: 15 minutes   **Servings**: 2

Ingredients:
- ➢ 1 package Gorton's Roasted Garlic
- ➢ Butter Grilled Tilapia (2 fillets)

1 can Gluten Free Soup (Try Amy's Organics or Roasted Red Pepper Tomato Soup)

Directions:
- ➢ Add two grilled fish fillets to a medium sized saucepan. Pour in 1 can (18.5oz) of Gluten Free Soup.
- ➢ Simmer until fish easily breaks into pieces. Stir often

24. SALADE NICOISE WITH LEMON VINAIGRETTE

Preparation Time: 20 minutes   **Cooking Time**: 15 minutes   **Servings**: 4

Ingredients:

SALAD
- ➢ Mixed greens
- ➢ Canned chunk tuna
- ➢ Hard boiled eggs
- ➢ Green beans Asparagus
- ➢ Cherry tomatoes
- ➢ Baby potatoes Kalamata olives Capers

DRESSING
- ➢ 2½ tsp GF grainy Dijon mustard
- ➢ ½ tsp honey
- ➢ ½ tsp dried tarragon Zest from half a lemon
- ➢ ¼ tsp salt
- ➢ ⅛ tsp pepper
- ➢ 3 drops GF Tabasco
- ➢ 2 Tbsp lemon juice or white wine vinegar
- ➢ 6 Tbsp olive oil

Directions:
- ➢ For the salad, boil eggs and potatoes until tender; remove from heat and set to one side.
- ➢ Steam asparagus and beans until tender-crisp.
- ➢ Submerge at once in cold water to stop the cooking process. Set to one side. Vegetables will be served at room temp.
- ➢ For the dressing, in a medium-size bowl place every ingredient except oil.
- ➢ Whisk and gradually drizzle in oil until all items are thick and well blended.

- ➢ (Do not use all the oil unless needed; stop when the thickness is right for you.)
- ➢ Taste dressing, then make any adjustments if necessary.
- ➢ On a large platter arrange pickled condiments, sliced eggs and vegetables, making it easy for everybody to select what they want.
- ➢ Put tongs beside platter; pour dressing into a gravy boat

25. BEAN SALAD

Preparation Time: 10 minutes **Cooking Time:** 0 minutes **Servings:** 4

Ingredients:

FOR THE SALAD:
- 16 ounces cooked kidney beans
- 3 cups cooked basmati rice
- 15 ounces cooked black beans
- 1/4 cup minced cilantro
- 1 1/2 cups frozen corn, thawed
- 4 green onions, sliced
- 1 small sweet red pepper, chopped

FOR THE DRESSING:
- ½ teaspoon minced garlic
- 1 teaspoon red chili powder
- 1 teaspoon salt
- 1/4 teaspoon ground black pepper
- 1 teaspoon ground cumin
- 1 tablespoon coconut sugar
- 1/2 cup olive oil
- 1/4 cup apple cider vinegar

Directions:
- Prepare the dressing and for this, place all its ingredients in a small bowl and whisk until combined.
- Place all the ingredients For the salad in another bowl, drizzle with salad dressing and toss until well coated.
- Portion the salad evenly between four salad mason jars and tighten with lid.
- Store the salad in the refrigerator for up to three days and serve

26. FENNEL IN TOMATO SAUCE

Preparation Time: 10 minutes **Cooking Time:** 25 minutes **Servings:** 4

Ingredients:
- 4 fennel bulbs
- 800 g tomatoes (peeled and deseeded)
- Parmesan cheese (grated)
- 1 red onion (chopped)
- 2 garlic cloves (crushed) white wine
- Black pepper
- Olive oil Method

Directions:
- Cut each fennel bulb lengthways into six wedges. Heat olive oil in a large frying pan over a medium heat.
- Add the fennel and cook for 5 minutes or until golden brown. Transfer the fennel over to a plate and leave to stand
- Then olive oil to the same frying pan and heat over a medium heat. Add the onion and garlic and cook for 2 minutes stirring continuously
- Join also a glass of white wine and cook for another minute. Add the tomatoes and fennel and cook for 25 minutes on a low heat
- Season with black pepper and parmesan cheese

27. HEARTY TOMATO SOUP

Preparation Time: 15 minutes **Cooking Time:** 6 H **Servings:** 6

Ingredients:
- 4 cups diced fresh tomatoes
- 4 cups natural chicken stock
- 2 celery stalks, diced
- 1 tablespoon chopped basil
- 2 carrots, peeled and diced 1 onion, chopped
- 1 cup heavy cream
- 2 teaspoons sea salt
- ½ cup grated Parmesan cheese

Directions:
- Place the tomatoes, chicken broth, celery, carrots and onion inside the slow cooker. Cover the pot and cook the tomato mixture for 5 hours on high temperature.
- Once the vegetables are tender, pour the contents of the slow cooker into a blender but do pass it through a strainer. Discard the remaining solids and puree the tomato mixture until it becomes smooth.
- Pour the pureed tomato mixture back into the slow cooker then mix in the cream, salt and basil. Cover the pot and cook the soup for another hour.
- Once the soup is ready, pour it into a serving bowl and top it with the grated Parmesan cheese

28. CHICKEN SOUP FOR THE GLUTEN-FREE SOUL

Preparation Time: 20 minutes   **Cooking Time**: 5 H   **Servings:**4

Ingredients:
- 4 chicken breasts, rinsed and dried
- 7 garlic cloves, minced
- 1 tablespoon olive oil
- 8 baby potatoes, sliced
- 2 zucchinis, peeled and diced
- 1 yellow bell pepper, deseeded and diced
- 1 yellow summer squash, peeled and diced
- 2 cups shredded cabbage
- 2 medium tomatoes, diced 1 teaspoon oregano
- 1 teaspoon dried basil
- 1 teaspoon chopped fresh parsley
- 3 cups natural chicken broth
- 1 teaspoon balsamic vinegar
- ½ teaspoon honey
- Salt and pepper to taste

Directions:
- Drizzle the olive oil inside the crock pot then place the chicken breasts inside
- Sprinkle some salt, pepper and the minced garlic on top of the chicken. Set this aside.
- In a separate bowl, mix together the potatoes, zucchinis, tomatoes, bell pepper, summer squash, cabbage, oregano, basil and parsley
- Toss the vegetables with the spices then add in the balsamic vinegar, honey and a sprinkle of salt and pepper.
- Pour the mixed vegetables on top of the chicken breasts then add in the chicken broth.
- Cover the pot lace the temperature on high. Cook the soup for 5 H or until the chicken is very tender

29. SPICY EGGPLANT STEW

Preparation Time: 15 minutes   **Cooking Time**: 8 H   **Servings:**8

Ingredients:
- ½ cup fresh vegetable stock
- 1 ½ cup pureed tomatoes
- garlic cloves, minced
- 2 ½ cups diced eggplant
- 1 cup chopped red onion
- 1 ½ cups diced zucchini 1 large tomato, chopped
- 1 ½ cups diced butternut squash
- 1 medium carrot, peeled and julienned
- 3 pieces frozen okra
- ¼ teaspoon paprika
- ¼ teaspoon chili powder
- ½ teaspoon cumin powder
- ½ teaspoon turmeric powder
- ½ teaspoon ground black pepper
- ½ teaspoon salt

Directions:
- Place the vegetable stock and pureed tomatoes inside the slow cooker
- Add in the eggplant, garlic, onion, zucchini, tomato, butternut squash, carrot and okra and mix.
- Then in all the spices into the stew and mix well. Cover the pot and set the temperature to low
- Cook the stew for 8 hours or until the vegetables are soft
- Pour the eggplant stew into a large soup bowl before serving

30. SLOW-COOKED CHILI CON CARNE

Preparation Time: 15 minutes   **Cooking Time**: 6 H   **Servings:**6

Ingredients:
- 450 grams ground beef
- 1 cup beef stock
- 1 teaspoon chili powder
- 1 teaspoon paprika
- 2 teaspoons cinnamon powder
- 1 red bell pepper, deseeded and diced
- 2 cups diced tomatoes
- 1 yellow onion, chopped
- 2 garlic cloves, minced
- 2 cups pureed pumpkin
- 1 cup diced green chilies

Directions:
- Place the ground beef in the slow cooker and set the temperature to low.
- Add in the beef stock, chili powder, paprika and cinnamon powder into the slow cooker and mix
- Stir in the bell pepper, tomatoes, onion, garlic, pureed pumpkin and green chilies.
- Cover the pot and cook the chili for 6 hours

31. BEEF & BEAN CASSEROLE

Preparation Time: 20 minutes   **Cooking Time**: 40 minutes   **Servings**: 6

Ingredients:
- Ground Beef (1 lb.)
- Chopped onion (.5 cup)
- Mushroom/chicken soup (1 cup)
- Salt (1 tsp.)
- Garlic powder (1/8 tsp.)
- Frozen green beans (16 oz.)
- Shredded cheddar cheese (as desired)
- GF tater tots (8 oz.)

Directions:
- Warm the oven to reach 350° Fahrenheit.
- Cook and drain the beans.
- Prepare the onion and beef in a skillet and drain the fat.
- Add the soup in a saucepan with the garlic and salt. Mix and add the onions and beef.
- Enjoy it for lunch or dinner. You can also use veggie crumbles instead of the meat for a change of pace!
- Dump it into a two-quart dish, adding half of the beans in the bottom with a layer of meat, cheese, beans, and beef
- Top it off with the tater tots.
- Bake the casserole for about 30 minutes and serve.

32. QUINOA AND BLACK BEAN STUFFED PEPPERS

Preparation Time: 15 minutes   **Cooking Time**: 20 minutes   **Servings**: 4

Ingredients:
- 4 large green bell peppers
- 1 cup quinoa, uncooked
- 15 ounces cooked black beans
- 1/2 cup ricotta cheese
- 2 cups tomato salsa
- 1/2 cup shredded Monterey Jack cheese
- 1 1/2 cups water

Directions:
- Switch on the oven, then set it to 400 degrees F, and let preheat.
- Take a small saucepan, place it over medium heat, pour in water, bring it boil
- Then add quinoa, reduce heat to medium-low level and simmer for 10 minutes until the quinoa has absorbed all the liquid.
- Meanwhile, prepare the peppers and for this, cut the peppers from the top, and remove seeds from them.
- Take an 8 inches baking dish, grease it with oil, place peppers in it cut side down and microwave for 4 minutes until tender-crisp.
- When quinoa has cooked, fluff it with a fork
- Then add 1 2/3 cups salsa along with ¼ cup Jack cheese, ricotta cheese, and beans and stir until well combined.
- Turn the bell pepper in the baking pan, cut side up, then stuff with the quinoa mixture
- Sprinkle remaining Jack cheese on top of stuffed peppers, and bake for 15 minutes.
- Let the peppers cool completely, then portion between four heatproof glass meal prep containers, tighten the container with lid
- Store in the refrigerator for up to one week or freeze for up to two months.
- When ready to eat, thaw the peppers, then reheat in the microwave
- until hot, top with remaining salsa and serve

33. MOROCCAN CHICKPEA QUINOA SALAD

Preparation Time: 10 minutes   **Cooking Time**: 22 minutes   **Servings**: 2

Ingredients:
- 15 ounces cooked chickpeas
- 1 cup quinoa, uncooked
- 1 medium white onion, peeled, diced
- ⅔ cup dried cranberries
- ⅓ cup diced parsley
- ½ teaspoon cumin
- ¼ teaspoon ground black pepper
- 1/2 teaspoon salt
- ½ teaspoon cinnamon
- 1 teaspoon ground turmeric
- ½ tablespoon coconut oil
- 2 cups vegetarian broth
- ½ cup sliced toasted almonds

Directions:
- Take a large pot, place it over medium heat, add oil and when hot, add onion and cook for 5 minutes until sauté.
- Then season with salt, black pepper, cumin, turmeric, and cinnamon and continue cooking for 30 seconds until fragrant.
- Add quinoa into the pot, pour in the broth, stir well and bring the mixture to boil.
- Then reduce heat to the low level and simmer the quinoa for 15 minutes until all the liquid is absorbed, covering the pot
- Remove the pot from heat, let it rest for 5 minutes, then fluff the quinoa with a fork, add chickpeas, parsley and cranberries and stir until well combined.
- Let the salad cool completely, then evenly portion between four salad mason jars and top with almonds.
- Tighten the jars with lid and refrigerate the salad for up to three days.
- Serve straight away

34. SWEET POTATO AND LENTIL SALADS

Preparation Time: 15 minutes   **Cooking Time**: 25 minutes   **Servings**: 4

Ingredients:

FOR THE VINAIGRETTE:
- 1 tablespoon minced garlic
- 1/2 teaspoon red chili powder
- 1/4 teaspoon salt
- 2 teaspoons honey
- 2 teaspoons lime juice
- 2 tablespoons apple cider vinegar
- 2 tablespoons olive oil

FOR THE SALAD:
- 19 ounces cooked brown lentils
- 6 cups sweet potato cubes
- 1 red bell pepper, sliced
- 11.5 ounces cooked corn kernels
- 1/2 teaspoon red chili powder
- 1 tablespoon olive oil

Directions:
- Switch on the oven, then set it to 425 degrees F, and let preheat.
- Prepare the vinaigrette and for this, place all its ingredients in a shaker and shake until well combined, set aside until required.
- Take a baking sheet, place sweet potato on it, drizzle with oil, toss until well coated
- Season with red chili powder and bake for 25 minutes until roasted, stirring halfway through, and when done, the sweet potato cubes cool completely.
- Assemble the salad and for this, spoon 1 tablespoon of prepared vinaigrette in four salad mason jars
- Then add ½ cup cooked lentils into each jar, top with ½ cup corn, 1 cup sweet potato, and slices of red bell pepper.
- Tighten the mason jars with lid and store in the refrigerator for up to four days

35. ORANGE TOFU CHICKPEA BOWLS

Preparation Time: 10 minutes   **Cooking Time:** 15 minutes   **Servings:**4

Ingredients:

- 14 ounces tofu, pressed, drained, cubed
- 6 cups broccoli florets, steamed
- 2 cups cooked brown rice
- 12 ounces cooked chickpeas
- 2 teaspoons sesame oil
- 1 tablespoon tamari
- 2 teaspoons sesame seeds

FOR THE ORANGE SAUCE:

- ½ teaspoon minced garlic
- 2 tablespoons maple syrup
- 1/2 teaspoon grated ginger
- 2 teaspoons cornstarch
- 2 tablespoons tamari
- 2 tablespoons toasted sesame oil
- 1/2 cup orange juice, unsweetened
- 1/4 cup water

Directions:

- Prepare the sauce and for this, place all its ingredients in a small bowl and whisk until well combined.
- Take a large skillet pan, place it over medium heat, add sesame oil and when hot, add tofu
- Drizzle with tamari and cook for 7 to 10 minutes until nicely browned.
- Then add chickpeas, pour in orange juice, stir well
- Cook for 3 minutes until the sauce has thickened enough to coat the back of a spoon, let cool completely.

- For meal prep, evenly portion rice between four heatproof glass
- meal prep containers, then add ¼ of the steamed broccoli into each container
- Top with ¼ of orange tofu and chickpeas, drizzle with extra sauce and garnish with sesame seeds.
- Tighten the containers with lid and refrigerate for up to five days or freeze for up to one month.
- When ready to eat, reheat the container in the microwave until hot and serve

36. TOFU STIR FRY

Preparation Time: 15 minutes   **Cooking Time:** 28 minutes   **Servings:**2

Ingredients:

- 1 bunch of baby bok choy, rinsed
- 1 ½ cups cooked brown rice
- 14 ounces tofu, pressed, drained, cubed
- 1 medium head of broccoli, chopped
- 3 medium carrots, peeled, chopped
- ½ teaspoon ground black pepper
- 1 teaspoon salt

- 3 tablespoons olive oil
- 1 teaspoon soy sauce
- 1 tablespoon water

FOR THE PEANUT SAUCE:

- ½ teaspoon minced garlic 1/4 cup honey
- 1/4 cup soy sauce
- 1 teaspoon apple cider vinegar 1/4 cup peanut butter
- 1 teaspoon sesame oil

Directions:

- Switch on the oven, then set it to 400 degrees F, and let it preheat in a large bowl and whisk until combined.
- Add tofu cubes in the sauce, toss until well coated and set aside.
- Take a large skillet pan, place it over medium heat, add 1 tablespoon oil and when hot, add bok choy
- Season with salt and black pepper and cook for 5 minutes.
- Then portion bok choy into three heatproof glass meal prep containers and set aside until required.
- Add 1 tablespoon oil in the pan, add broccoli and carrot, sprinkle with black pepper
- Drizzle with soy sauce and water, stir well and cook for 7 minutes, covering the pan.

- Then portion the vegetables into meal prep containers containing bok choy and set aside until required.
- Add remaining oil into the skillet pan, add tofu pieces in it
- Cook for 10 minutes until nicely browned, flipping the tofu every 3 minutes.
- Take a baking sheet, line it with aluminum foil, spread tofu pieces on it, and bake for 5 minutes.
- Add ½ cup cooked brown rice into each meal prep container
- Then top with tofu, let cool completely, and then tighten the container with lid.
- Store the meal prep container in the refrigerator for up to four days or freeze for up to two months.
- When ready to eat, reheat the container in the microwave until hot and serve

37. COD AND VEGGIES

Preparation Time: 10 minutes   **Cooking Time**: 25 minutes   **Servings**:4

Ingredients:

➢ 1 pound cod, cut into 4 pieces
➢ 2 cups cherry tomatoes
➢ 2 cups diced purple potatoes
➢ 1 teaspoon dried thyme

➢ 1 ½ teaspoon salt
➢ 1 teaspoon ground black pepper
➢ 1 teaspoon garlic powder
➢ 4 tablespoons olive oil

Directions:

➢ Switch on the oven, then set it to 400 degrees F, and let it preheat.
➢ Take a baking sheet, spread potatoes on it, drizzle with 2 tablespoons oil, toss until well coated, and roast for 15 minutes.
➢ Then add push tomatoes to one side of the sheet, add cod and tomatoes
➢ Drizzle remaining oil over them, season with black pepper, salt, thyme, and garlic powder

➢ Then continue baking for 10 minutes until thoroughly cooked.
➢ Let the salmon, potatoes, and tomatoes cool and then portion evenly between four heatproof meal prep containers.
➢ Tighten the containers with lid and store in the refrigerator for up to four days or freeze for up to one month.
➢ When ready to eat, thaw the fish and vegetables, then reheat in a microwave until hot and serve

38. GRILLED VEGETABLE AND BLACK BEAN BOWLS

Preparation Time: 15 minutes   **Cooking Time**: 15 minutes   **Servings**:4

Ingredients:

FOR THE VINAIGRETTE:
➢ 1/4 teaspoon salt
➢ 1/4 teaspoon red chili powder
➢ 2 teaspoons honey
➢ 1 tablespoons apple cider vinegar
➢ 3 tablespoons BBQ sauce
➢ 1 teaspoon lime juice

FOR THE MEAL PREP BOWLS:
➢ 2 cups cooked quinoa
➢ 18 ounces cooked black beans
➢ 1 medium zucchini, chopped
➢ ½ of medium red onion, peeled, chopped
➢ 2 medium red bell peppers, chopped
➢ 2/3 teaspoon ground black pepper
➢ 1 teaspoon salt
➢ 1 tablespoon olive oil

Directions:

➢ Prepare the vinaigrette, and for this, place all its ingredients in a shaker and shale until well combined, set aside until required.
➢ Place zucchini, onion and bell pepper in a large bowl, drizzle with oil, season with black pepper and salt, and toss until well coated.
➢ Take a grill pan, place it over medium heat, grease it with oil and when hot

➢ Arrange vegetables on it and grill for 10 to 15 minutes until cooked, flipping every 5 minutes.
➢ For meal prep, portion quinoa into four heatproof glass meal prep containers, top evenly with grilled vegetables and black pepper, and then drizzle with vinaigrette generously.
➢ Tighten the meal prep containers with lid and store in the refrigerator for up to four days or freeze for up to two months.
➢ When ready to eat, reheat the container in the microwave until hot, and serve

39. SALAD WITH CHICKPEAS AND TUNA

Preparation Time: 10 minutes   **Cooking Time**: 0 minutes   **Servings**:1

Ingredients:

➢ 2.5-ounce tuna, pouched
➢ ½ cup cooked chickpeas
➢ 3 cups chopped kale

➢ Transfer kale into a 1-quart mason jar
➢ 1 medium carrot, peeled and shredded
➢ 2 tablespoons honey-mustard vinaigrette

Directions:

➢ Cut kale into bite-size pieces, add them in a bowl, then add vinaigrette and toss until well coated.

➢ Top with chickpeas, tuna, and carrot and tighten the jar with lid.
➢ Refrigerate the jar for up to two days and serve

40. SHRIMP AVOCADO SALAD

Preparation Time: 10 minutes   **Cooking Time:** 0 minutes   **Servings:**6

Ingredients:

FOR THE SALAD:
- ➤ 1 pound shrimp, peeled, deveined, cooked, chopped
- ➤ 1/4 cup chopped red onion
- ➤ 2 plum tomatoes, seeded, chopped
- ➤ 1 jalapeno pepper, deseeded, minced
- ➤ 2 green onions, chopped
- ➤ 1 serrano pepper, deseeded, minced
- ➤ 2 tablespoons minced fresh cilantro

FOR THE DRESSING:
- ➤ 1 teaspoon adobo seasoning
- ➤ 2 tablespoons apple cider vinegar
- ➤ 2 tablespoons lime juice
- ➤ 2 tablespoons olive oil
- ➤ FOR SERVING:
- ➤ 3 medium avocados, peeled and cubed
- ➤ 12 big lettuce leaves
- ➤ 6 wedges of lime

Directions:
- ➤ Place all the ingredients for the salad in a large bowl and toss until just mixed.
- ➤ Prepare the dressing and for this, place all its ingredients in a small bowl and whisk until combined.
- ➤ Drizzle the dressing over the salad, toss until well coated, and then stir in avocado.
- ➤ Portion two lettuce leaves into six heatproof glass meal prep containers, then top evenly with prepared salad.
- ➤ Add a lime wedge into each container, then tighten the containers with lid and store in the refrigerator for up to three days.
- ➤ Serve straight away as a wrap

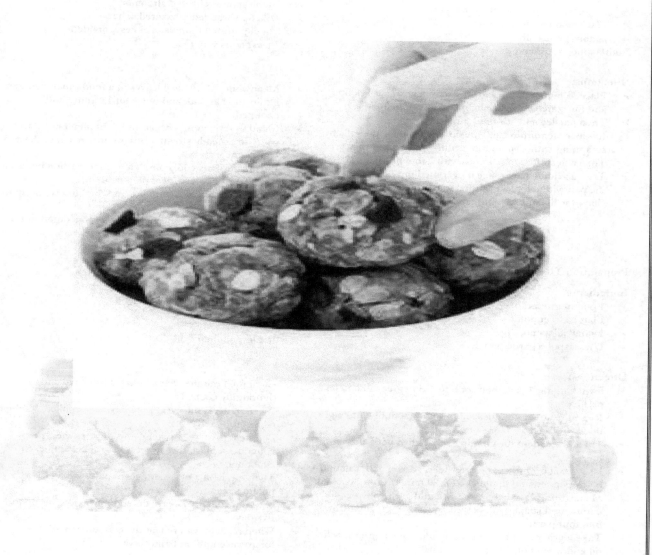

41. STUFFED PORTOBELLO MUSHROOMS

Preparation Time: 10 minutes   **Cooking Time:** 10 minutes   **Servings:** 2

Ingredients:
- 6 large portobello mushrooms
- 6 slices of a large tomato
- 1/8 teaspoon ground black pepper
- ½ teaspoon minced garlic
- 2 tablespoons olive oil

2 tablespoons minced parsley

- 3/4 cup fresh basil leaves
- 3/4 cup ricotta cheese
- 2 tablespoons slivered almonds
- 1/2 cup shredded mozzarella cheese
- 3/4 cup grated Parmesan cheese, divided
- 3 teaspoons water

Directions:
- Place ¼ cup of parmesan cheese in a bowl, add ricotta and mozzarella cheese along with black pepper
- Then parsley and stir until mixed.
- Remove stem from each mushroom, remove the gills by scrapping with a spoon, then stuff with cheese mixture
- Top each stuffed mushroom with a tomato slice.
- Take a griddle pan, place it over medium heat, grease the pan with oil, place stuffed mushrooms on it
- Cook for 10 minutes until tender.

- Meanwhile, place basil leaves in a food processor, add garlic and almond, and pulse for 1 minute until chopped.
- Blend in remaining cheese and then blend in oil and water in a steady stream until mixture reach to desired consistency.
- Let mushrooms cool completely, then portion between two heatproof glass meal prep containers
- Cover the containers with lid, and then freeze for up to one month.
- When ready to eat, reheat the mushrooms until hot, then top with cheese mixture and serve

42. JALAPENO SLIDERS

Preparation Time: 10 minutes   **Cooking Time:** 200 minutes   **Servings:** 2

Ingredients:
- 1 pound ground beef
- 1 large sweet potato
- 1 small jalapeno, diced
- 1/2 teaspoon garlic powder

- 2/3 teaspoon ground black pepper
- 1/2 teaspoon cumin
- 1 teaspoon salt
- 1tablespoon olive oil

Directions:
- Switch on the oven, then set it to 425 degrees F, and let it preheat.
- Rinse the sweet potatoes, cut into horizontally into eight thick slices
- Then place them on a baking sheet lined with aluminum foil.
- Drizzle oil over sweet potato slices, season with salt and black pepper, and then bake for 20 minutes until cooked.
- Meanwhile, place beef in a bowl, add garlic powder, cumin, and jalapeno, mix well and shape the mixture into four patties.
- Take a grill pan, place it over medium heat, grease with oil and when hot, add patties on it

- Cook for 4 minutes per side until browned and thoroughly cooked.
- When patties and sweet potatoes have cooked, let them cool completely.
- For meal prep, take two heatproof glass meal prep containers, place two sweet potato slices into each container
- Then top with a patty and cover patty with a sweet potato slice.
- Shut the containers with lid and refrigerate for up to five days.
- When ready to eat, reheat the containers in the microwave until hot and serve

43. PEANUT BUTTER ENERGY BITES

Preparation Time: 40 minutes   **Cooking Time:** 0 minutes   Servings:18

Ingredients:
- 2 tablespoons ground flax
- 1 1/2 cups rolled oats
- 1/4 cup chia seeds
- 2 tablespoons cocoa powder, unsweetened
- 1/2 cup protein powder
- 2 tablespoons agave syrup
- 1/2 cup peanut butter
- 1 cup water

Directions:
- Place chia seeds in a bowl, pour in water, stir in protein powder, stir until mixed and refrigerate for 5 minutes.
- Then place remaining ingredients in another bowl, add chia seeds mixture
- Stir until well combined and then with a wet hand, shape the mixture into 1-inch balls, about eighteen.
- Place balls on a sheet pan lined with parchment paper and freeze for 30 minutes until firm.
- Store the energy balls in the refrigerator for up to one week
- (Or transfer them into a freezer-proof bag and freeze for up to one month)

44. THAI TURKEY LETTUCE WRAPS

Preparation Time: 10 minutes   **Cooking Time:** 10 minutes   Servings:6

Ingredients:
FOR THE SAUCE:
- 3 tablespoons soy sauce
- 1 tablespoon lime juice
- 2 tablespoons rice vinegar
- 1/4 cup peanut butter
- 1 teaspoon sesame oil
- 2 tablespoons water
- FOR THE FILLING:
- 1 pound ground turkey
- 1 medium white onion, peeled, chopped
- 1 cup shredded carrots
- 1 tablespoon minced garlic
- 1 tablespoon Thai red curry paste

1 tablespoon olive oil
FOR SERVING:
- Green onions as needed to garnish
- 7 ounces Romaine lettuce leaf
- Peanuts as needed to garnish

Directions:
- Prepare the sauce and for this, place all the ingredients For the sauce in a bowl
- Whisk well until combined, and set aside until required.
- Prepare the filling and for this, take a skillet pan, place it over medium heat, add oil and when hot, add garlic, onion and curry paste, stir well and cook for 3 minutes until heated.
- Then add turkey, break it up, stir well and continue cooking for 7 minutes until turkey is no longer pink and thoroughly cooked.
- Add carrots and peanut sauce, stir until mixed, and then remove the pan from heat.
- For meal prep, let the turkey mixture cool completely and then evenly portion between six heatproof glass meal prep containers.
- Cover the containers with a lid, store them in the refrigerator for up to four days or freeze for up to one month.
- When ready to eat, thaw the frozen turkey mixture and then reheat in the microwave oven until hot.
- Stuff the turkey mixture in lettuce leaves, top with green onions and peanuts, and serve

45. CHIPOTLE HONEY CHICKEN TACO SALAD

Preparation Time: 10 minutes   **Cooking Time**: 4 H   **Servings:**4

Ingredients:

FOR THE CHICKEN:
- 2 chicken breasts
- ½ teaspoon minced garlic
- 1/4 teaspoon salt
- 1/4 cup honey
- 1 tablespoon lime juice
- 2 tablespoons adobo sauce
- 1/4 cup chicken stock

FOR THE SALAD:
- 1 medium green bell pepper, sliced
- 2 medium carrots, peeled, shredded
- 3 cups shredded cabbage

FOR SERVING:
- Tortilla chips as needed

Directions:
- Prepare the chicken and for this, place chicken in a slow cooker, add remaining ingredients and toss until well coated.
- Switch on the slow cooker, shut it with lid
- Cook for 4 hours at low heat setting or for 3 hours at high heat setting until chicken is tender, don't overcook.
- Let the chicken cool completely, then evenly divide it between four glass meal prep containers and drizzle with sauce.
- Cover the containers with the lid, store them in the refrigerator for up to four days or freeze for up to one month
- When ready to eat, thaw the frozen chicken and then reheat in the microwave oven until hot.
- Let chicken cool slightly, then add the ingredients For the salad and toss until mixed.
- Top the chicken salad with tortilla chips and serve

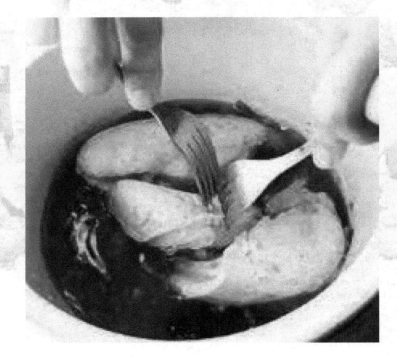

46. SWEET POTATO, LENTIL, AND KALE SALAD

Preparation Time: 10 minutes   **Cooking Time**: 35 minutes   **Servings:4**

Ingredients:

FOR THE SALAD:
- 3/4 cup brown lentils, uncooked
- 4 cups cubed sweet potato, peeled
- 2 teaspoons olive oil
- 4 cups chopped kale
- 1 large red bell pepper, cored, diced
- 1/4 cup diced red onion
- 3 teaspoons salt
- 1 teaspoon ground black pepper
- ¼ cup roasted pumpkin seeds
- 1 ½ cup water

FOR THE TAHINI DRESSING:
- 1/3 cup tahini
- ½ tablespoon minced garlic
- 1/4 teaspoon salt
- 1/2 teaspoon curry powder
- 2 tablespoons lemon juice
- 7 tablespoons water

Directions:

- Switch on the oven, then set it to 375 degrees F and let preheat.
- Take a large sheet pan, add sweet potato cubes on it, drizzle with oil
- Then sprinkle with 1 ½ teaspoon salt and black pepper
- Toss until mixed and bake for 35 minutes until tender, stirring halfway through.
- Meanwhile, prepare the lentils and for this, take a mediumsaucepan
- Place it over medium heat, pour in water, add lentils and ½ teaspoon salt, bring it to simmer
- Cook for 20 minutes until lentils are tender, let cool completely.
- Prepare the dressing and for this, place all its ingredients in a bowl

- Whisk until combined, set aside until required.
- Prepare kale and for this, place kale in a bowl, season with remaining salt, drizzle with lemon juice
- Then massage the kale leaves for 30 seconds until slightly softened and set aside.
- Assemble the salad and for this, take four mason jars, spoon 2 tablespoons of prepared dressing in the bottom of each jar
- Then add ½ cup of cooked lentils
- Top with ½ cup baked sweet potato and ¼ of diced red peppers, and then add 1 tablespoon onion and 1 cup kale leaves.
- Prepare three more mason salad jars in the same manner, then tighten with lid and refrigerate for four days.
- When ready to eat, top the salad with a tablespoon of pumpkin seeds and serve

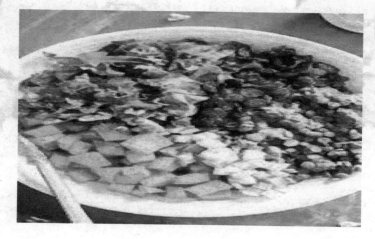

47. PEANUT-LIME CHICKEN BOWL

Preparation Time: 30 minutes   **Cooking Time**: 30 minutes   **Servings:4**

Ingredients:

FOR THE RICE:
- 3/4 cup brown rice, uncooked
- 3/4 cup chicken stock
- 3/4 cup water 1/4 teaspoon salt
- 1 tablespoon lime zest

FOR THE CHICKEN:
- 16 ounces chicken breasts
- 1 tablespoon olive oil
- 1 tablespoon soy sauce

FOR THE VEGETABLES:
- 2 cups diced carrots
- 2 cups broccoli florets
- 1 tablespoon olive oil

FOR THE PEANUT LIME SAUCE:
- 1/4 cup peanut butter
- 1 1/2 tablespoons apple cider vinegar
- 1/2 tablespoon brown sugar
- 1/2 teaspoon sesame oil
- 1/2 tablespoon lime juice
- 2 tablespoons of water or more as needed to thin it out

FOR SERVING
- 1/4 cup peanuts

Directions:

- Switch on the oven, then set it to 425 degrees F, and let preheat.
- Cook the rice and for this, place a saucepan over medium-high heat, add all the ingredients for rice, stir well and bring it to boil.
- Then reduce heat to medium-low level
- Simmer rice for 20 minutes or more until the rice has absorbed all the liquid and tender
- Fluff the cooked rice with a fork, and set aside.
- Prepare the chicken and for this, place chicken in a small baking pan
- Drizzle with oil and soy sauce, toss until well coated on both sides
- Then bake for 20 minutes until cooked through, flipping the chicken halfway.
- Meanwhile, take a large baking sheet, place carrot and broccoli florets on it, drizzle with oil
- Toss until well coated and bake the vegetables with chicken for 20 minutes until roasted, stirring halfway through.
- Prepare the sauce and for this, place peanut butter in a heatproof bowl, microwave for 30 seconds
- Then stir until smooth, add remaining ingredients for the sauce
- Whisk until well combined, whisk in 2 tablespoons water if the sauce is too thick.
- For meal prep, cool the chicken and vegetables, then divide them evenly between for glass meal prep containers
- Join also boiled rice and then drizzle 2 tablespoons of prepared sauce over chicken in each container.
- Cover the containers with the lid, store them in the refrigerator for up to five days or freeze for up to one month.
- When ready to eat, thaw the frozen chicken and vegetables, and then reheat in the microwave oven until hot.
- Sprinkle peanuts over chicken and serve

48. MEDITERRANEAN CHICKPEA SALAD

Preparation Time: 10 minutes   **Cooking Time**: 0 minutes   **Servings:6**

Ingredients:

FOR THE CHICKPEA SALAD:
- 1 cup cubed cucumber
- 1 1/2 cups chickpeas, cooked
- 1/2 cup chopped parsley leaves
- 1/2 of large red onion, peeled, chopped
- 1 cup cubed cherry tomatoes
- 1/4 cup feta cheese, crumbled

FOR THE VINAIGRETTE
- 1/4 teaspoon ground black pepper
- 1/2 teaspoon sea salt
- 1 teaspoon Dijon mustard
- 2 teaspoons lemon juice 1/4 cup olive oil
- 1 tablespoon apple cider vinegar

Directions:

- Place all the ingredients For the salad in a bowl and toss until just mixed.
- Prepare the vinaigrette and for this, place all its ingredients in another bowl and whisk until combined.
- Drizzle with vinaigrette over chickpea salad, toss until well mixed and then portion it between three meal prep containers.
- Tighten the containers with lid and store in the refrigerator for up to four days. Serve when ready.

49. ALMOND BUTTER TURKEY MEATBALLS

Preparation Time: 10 minutes   **Cooking Time**: 12 minutes   Servings:4

Ingredients:

FOR THE MEATBALLS:
- 1 pond ground turkey breast
- 1 teaspoon garlic powder
- 1 teaspoon onion powder
- ½ teaspoon ground ginger

FOR PEANUT BUTTER SAUCE:
- 2 tablespoons red curry paste 1 tablespoon coconut sugar
- 1/2 cup almond butter
- 1 tablespoon soy sauce
- 1 tablespoon apple cider vinegar
- 4 tablespoons lime juice
- 3/4 cup coconut milk

Directions:
- Switch on the oven, then set it to 425 degrees F, and let it preheat.
- Prepare the sauce and for this, place all its ingredients in a bowl and whisk until combined.
- Place all the ingredients for meatballs in another bowl, mix well and then shape the mixture into fourteen meatballs.
- Take a skillet pan, grease it with oil, spread ¼ cup of the sauce and then place meatballs in it.
- Top the meatballs with remaining sauce and bake for 12 minutes until meatballs have thoroughly cooked.
- Let meatballs cool completely
- Then pour the meatballs and sauce evenly between four heatproof glass meal prep containers and tighten with lid
- Store the containers in the refrigerator for up to four days or freeze for up to one month.
- When ready to eat, thaw the meatballs, then reheat in the microwave until hot and serve.

50. CHIPOTLE SHREDDED CHICKEN

Preparation Time: 10 minutes   **Cooking Time**: 30 minutes   Servings:4

Ingredients:
- 1 pound chicken breasts
- 3 chipotle peppers in adobo sauce, minced
- 1 ½ teaspoon minced garlic
- 1 teaspoon adobo sauce
- 1/2 cup chopped fresh cilantro
- 2 teaspoons yellow mustard
- 1 tablespoon olive oil
- 2 cups chicken broth
- 1 cup orange juice, unsweetened

Directions:
- Take a large pot, place it over medium heat, add oil and when hot, add garlic and chipotle pepper
- cook for 2 minutes until sauté, stirring continuously.
- Switch heat to the high level, add cilantro, pour in chicken broth and orange juice, stir well and bring the mixture to boil.
- Then add chicken, switch heat to medium-low level and simmer for 15 to 20 minutes until the chicken has thoroughly cooked.
- When done, transfer chicken to a cutting board, let it rest for 5 minutes, and then shred it with two forks.
- In the meantime, whisk mustard into the sauce and continue cooking the sauce over low heat until reduced by half.
- Return the shredded chicken into the pot, toss until well coated in sauce, and then let cool.
- For meal prep, divide chicken evenly between four glass meal prep containers, tighten them with lid
- Refrigerate for up to three days or freeze for up to one month.
- When ready to eat, thaw the chicken, then reheat in the microwave until hot and serve

51. FLOURLESS PEANUT BUTTER-CHOCOLATE CHIP COOKIES

Preparation Time: 20 minutes   **Cooking Time**: 20 minutes   **Servings**:2

Ingredients:
- 1 cup creamy peanut butter
- 3/4 cup sugar
- 1 large egg
- 1/2 teaspoon baking soda
- 1/4 teaspoon salt
- 1 cup semisweet chocolate morsels

Directions:
- Preheat oven to 350°F (180°C).
- Stir together peanut butter and next 4 ingredients in a medium bowl until well blended. Stir in chocolate morsels.
- Drop dough by rounded tablespoonfuls 2 inches apart onto parchment paper- lined baking sheets.
- Bake at 350°F (180°C)for 12 to 14 minutes or until puffed and lightly browned.
- Cool on baking sheets on a wire rack 5 minutes. Transfer to wire rack, and let cool 15 minutes

52. NO BAKE TIRAMISU COOKIES

Preparation Time: 20 minutes   **Cooking Time**: 40 minutes   **Servings**:15

Ingredients:
- 1 cup gluten free oat flour (gluten free oats ground to a flour)
- 1 T cocoa powder
- 1 T espresso powder (or ground coffee powder)
- 1/4 tsp sea salt
- 1 scoop vanilla protein powder*
- 2 T granulated sweetener of choice (optional)
- 1/4 cup almond butter
- 1/4- 3/4 cup dairy free milk (I use Blue Diamond Unsweetened vanilla)
- Espresso powder, granulated sweetener of choice to dust

Directions:
- Combine the flour, cocoa powder, espresso powder, sea salt, protein powder in large bowl and stir until well mixed.
- Add almond butter; using two knives, cut into dry mixture till it's extremely crumbly.
- Put in a tablespoon of unsweetened vanilla milk at a time until you have an extremely dense dough.
- Form into palm sized cookie shapes with your hands, then press densely on your platter
- Dust the granulated sweetener, espresso and rest of cocoa. For a softer cookie, consume now
- For a denser cookie, put in refrigerator a minimum of 10 minutes

53. BACON-WRAPPED FIGS

Preparation Time:10 minutes   **Cooking Time**: 20 minutes   **Servings**:4

Ingredients:
- Figs (12)
- Thin-cut bacon/pancetta (3-6 pieces)

Directions:
- Rinse and pat dry the figs. Remove any stems.
- Slice the bacon in half.
- Wrap each fig with a strip of bacon.
- Heat a large skillet using the med-high temperature setting.
- Cook them until each side is browned and crispy as desired.
- Place them on several layers of paper towels to drain the fat oils before serving them

54. BACON-WRAPPED JALAPENO POPPERS

Preparation Time: 10 minutes   **Cooking Time:** 35 minutes   **Servings:** 4

Ingredients:
- Jalapenos (12)
- Bacon (1 lb.)
- Cream/goat cheese (8 oz.)
- Balsamic glaze/ barbecue sauce (.25 cup)
- Garlic salt (as desired)

Directions:
- Set the oven at 425° Fahrenheit.
- Slice the jalapenos in half - lengthwise- and discard the pith and seeds. It's recommended to wear gloves during the process.
- Place the prepared jalapenos on a baking tray and fill them with cheese using a piping bag.
- Sprinkle them with the salt and wrap with ½ slice of bacon.
- Baste the tops with the sauce.
- Set a timer to bake them for 20 minutes until it's crispy to your liking

55. BUFFALO QUINOA BITES

Preparation Time: 10 minutes   **Cooking Time:** 50 minutes   **Servings:** 30

Ingredients:
- Cooked quinoa (2 cups)
- Eggs (4)
- Tomato paste (3 tbsp.)
- Sea salt - fine grain (1 tsp.)
- Garlic powder (.5 tsp.)
- Ground black pepper (.25 tsp.)
- Cayenne pepper (.5 tsp.)
- Paprika (.5 tsp.)
- Breadcrumbs (1 cup)
- Mozzarella (30 - ½-inch cubes)

THE SAUCE:
- Butter (½ stick or 4 oz.)
- Hot sauce Red Hot (.5 cup)

Directions:
- Warm the oven at 350°Fahrenheit. Cover a baking tray using a layer of parchment baking paper.
- Combine/whisk the eggs, tomato paste, quinoa, garlic powder, salt, black pepper, and paprika into a mixing container.
- Mix in the breadcrumbs and wait two to three minutes.
- Scoop one heaping tablespoon of the quinoa mixture to make the quinoa balls
- Push a cube of mozzarella into the middle of the ball and close it
- Repeat the process until the mixture is gone, placing them on the prepared tray.
- Set the timer to bake for 15 minutes
- Mix the hot sauce and butter in a saucepan using the medium-temperature setting
- Remove the baking tray from the oven and top with buffalo sauce.
- Bake them for another eight minutes.
- Serve with celery sticks and blue cheese dip as desired

56. CHEESY MASHED POTATO BALLS

Preparation Time: 15 minutes   **Cooking Time**: 355 minutes   Servings:3

Ingredients:
- Mashed potato (2 boiled)
- Spring onions (2 tbsp.)
- Coriander leaves (2 tbsp.)
- Ginger (2 tsp.)
- Garlic (2 tsp.)
- Green chili (1)
- Coriander powder (1 tsp.)
- Chilli powder (2 tsp.)
- Garam masala (1 tsp.)
- Pepper (2 tsp.)
- Cumin powder (1 tsp.)
- Cheese (.5 cup)
- Salt (as desired)
- THE BATTER:
- Maida (.5 cup)
- Chilli powder (1 tsp.)
- Rice flour (2 tbsp.)
- Pepper (.5 tsp.)
- Water (1 cup)

Directions:
- Boil and peel the potatoes. Finely chop the green chili.
- Combine the cheese fixings with the potatoes and form them into balls. Leave them on a tray for now.
- Prepare the batter by combining the seasonings, flour, and maida in a mixing container
- Add water a little at a time, whisking to prevent it from being lumpy.
- Warm the oil in a wok.
- Dip the potato balls into the batter - one at a time - to fry them using the medium temperature setting.
- Remove them and drain on paper towels to serve

57. ESPINACAS A LA CATALANA

Preparation Time: 5 minutes   **Cooking Time**: 8 minutes   Servings:4

Ingredients:
- Spinach (2 cups)
- Cashews (3 tbsp.)
- Garlic cloves (2)
- Dried currants (3 tbsp.)
- Avocado or olive oil (as needed)

Directions:
- Peel and mince the garlic. Add a bit of oil into a skillet to heat (medium temp)
- Toss in the garlic to sauté for about one to two minutes.
- Rinse and snip the stems from the spinach and steam it for a few minutes.
- Fold in the currants and cashews to sauté for about one minute. Fold in the spinach.
- Toss it thoroughly with the oil and salt before serving

58. MACHO NACHOS

Preparation Time: 5 minutes   **Cooking Time**: 50 minutes   Servings:8

Ingredients:
- Lean ground beef (1 lb.)
- GF corn tortilla chips (12 oz.)
- GF taco seasoning (2 tbsp.)
- Grated Monterey Jack/Cheddar cheese (12 oz.)
- Red/orange Bell pepper (.5 cup - chopped)
- Sweet yellow onion (.5 cup - chopped)
- Sliced black olives (.5 cup - blot dry)
- Pickled Jalapeno peppers (.5 cup - blot dry)
- Green onions (.5 cup - thinly sliced)
- Roma tomatoes (.5 cup - chopped and blot dry)
- Fresh cilantro (.25 cup)
- Also Needed: 13 x 9-inch baking dish

Directions:
- Brown the beef in a cast-iron skillet. Drain the fat and stir in the taco seasoning. Set it aside for now.
- Set the oven at 400° Fahrenheit.
- Spread a layer of one-third of the corn chips in the baking dish.
- Add one-third of the cooked hamburger evenly over the chips.
- Lastly, sprinkle one-third of each (chopped jalapenos, yellow onions, bell pepper, green onions, black olives, and tomatoes) over the hamburger.
- Sprinkle one-third of a cup of shredded cheese over the vegetables.
- Continue with two more layers.
- Bake them until the cheese melts (20 min.).
- Serve with a sprinkle freshly chopped cilantro

59. SPINACH BALLS

Preparation Time: 10 minutes   **Cooking Time**: 25 minutes   **Servings:40 Balls**

Ingredients:
- Frozen chopped spinach (16 oz.)
- Butter (6 tbsp.)
- Eggs (3)
- Cheddar cheese (.75 cup - grated)
- Parmesan cheese (3 oz. - finely grated)
- Sweet paprika (.5 tsp.)
- Dry Italian spice mix (.5 tsp.)
- Fresh parsley (1/3 cup)
- Corn Chex cereal (4 cups/ finely crushed - 1.5 cups)
- GF flour (3 tbsp.)

Directions:
- Set the oven temperature at 350° Fahrenheit. Cover two baking trays with a layer of parchment baking paper.
- Thaw, chop the spinach and place it into a colander
- Use a wooden spoon to press the spinach and remove as much moisture as possible
- Twist it dry in a bunch of paper towels or a tea towel.
- Melt and add the butter and eggs in a bowl to beat until the mixture frothy
- Add in the cheeses, spices, and minced parsley, and spinach. Mix well
- Stir the flour and cereal, stirring until the clumps of spinach are removed.
- Scoop the mixture, rolling it in your hands to make the balls
- Put them onto the prepared baking trays and set the timer to bake for 15 minutes.
- Note: Measure the four cups of cereal and crush it to reach 1.5 cups of breadcrumbs

60. SPINACH & ARTICHOKE RISOTTO BALLS

Preparation Time: 10 minutes   **Cooking Time**: 60 minutes   **Servings:10**

Ingredients:
- GF Chicken broth (4 cups)
- Olive oil (2 tbsp.)
- Shallots (2 small or 1/3 cup)
- Garlic (2 cloves)
- Fine sea salt
- Arborio rice (1.5 cups)
- Dry white wine (.5 cup)
- Parmesan cheese - freshly grated (.5 cup)
- Artichoke hearts in olive oil (9.87 oz. jar)
- Fresh baby spinach (2 cups)
- GF flour (1 cup)
- Pepper & salt (to your liking)
- Eggs (2)
- Water (2 tsp.)
- GF Italian breadcrumbs (2 cups)
- Canola oil (as needed for frying)
  FOR SERVING:
- Marinara sauce
- Shaved parmesan cheese

Directions:
- Chop the shallots and mince the garlic. Drain and chop the artichoke hearts.
- Heat the chicken broth in a saucepan.
- Warm the olive oil in a large sauté pan using the medium temperature setting
- Once the pan is hot, toss in the shallots, garlic, pepper, and salt to sauté about three minutes.
- Pour in the rice to sauté an additional two to three minutes until the rice is toasted.
- Pour and stir the wine until it's almost evaporated.
- Pour in the broth (.5 cup at a time). After the rice absorbs it, add another half cupù
- Stir and let it finish cooking until it's firm or as desired (al dente).
- Fold in the spinach, artichokes, and grated parmesan
- Dump the risotto into a dish and place it in the fridge overnight.
- When it's chilled, roll it into two-inch balls (20).
- Set up three bowls;1 with flour, salt, and pepper; 2 - whisk the eggs and mix with water; 3 will have breadcrumbs.
- Simply, roll each of the balls in the flour, egg, and breadcrumbs until thoroughly coated
- Arrange them on a platter and continue until all are done. Pop them in the fridge for at least thirty minutes or overnight.
- Fry Time: Warm the about three inches of oil in a large, heavy- bottom pot to reach 375° Fahrenheit).
- Cook the risotto balls in batches until browned (2 min.). Remove and drain on paper towels
- (Pop them into a 200° Fahrenheit oven to keep warm.)
- Serve the balls hot. Garnish them using a portion of parmesan cheese and parsley. Enjoy with a warm marinara sauce for dipping

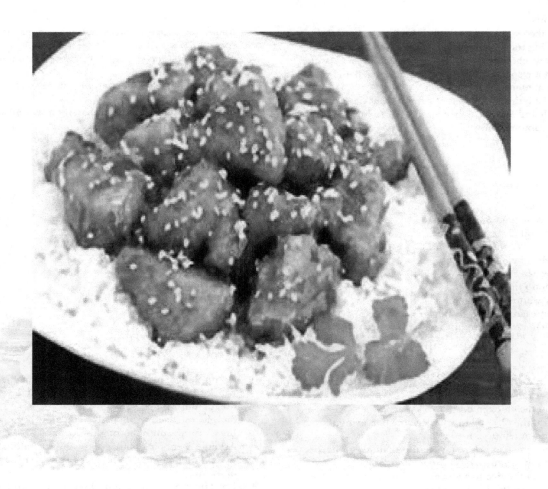

61. SLOW-COOKED SWEET HAM

Preparation Time: 5 minutes   **Cooking Time**: 6 H 30 minutes   Servings:8

Ingredients:
- 3 kg bone-in ham, unwrapped
- 3 cups pineapple juice
- 1 cup maple syrup
- ½ cup brown sugar

Directions:
- Place the ham in a large slow cooker. Rub the brown sugar on all sides of the meat.
- Pour the pineapple juice and maple syrup on top of the ham.
- Cover the pot and set the temperature to low.
- Cook for 7 hours or until the ham is tender once a fork is poked into it.
- Turn off the slow cooker and let the ham stand for 20 minutes.
- Remove the ham from the slow cooker and place it on a cutting board
- Cut a few slices of the ham and place it on a serving dish together with the whole meat. Pour the sauce over the meat before serving

62. SPICY HONEY SESAME CHICKEN

Preparation Time: 10 minutes   **Cooking Time**: 4 H   Servings:6

Ingredients:
- 1 pound boneless and skinless chicken breasts
- 1 tablespoon chili powder
- 3 tablespoons raw honey
- 2 teaspoons sesame oil
- 2 tablespoons pureed tomatoes
- 1 teaspoon chopped chilies
- 1 teaspoon sesame seeds
- 1 teaspoon chopped green onions
- ½ cup chopped yellow onion
- 2 tablespoons apple cider vinegar
- 3 tablespoons gluten-free soy sauce
- 2 tablespoons water
- 1 teaspoon minced garlic
- 2 teaspoons corn starch

Directions:
- Dissolve the corn starch in water until it is free of lumps. Set this aside.
- In a separate bowl, mix together the soy sauce, apple cider vinegar, sesame oil, honey, chili powder and pureed tomatoes
- Add in the yellow onions, garlic, chilies and chicken breasts and mix well.
- Place the chicken breasts inside the slow cooker and pour the sauce on top
- Cover the slow cooker and set the temperature to high. Cook for 4 hours or until the chicken is tender.
- Top with green onions and sesame seeds before serving

63. LAMB CURRY WITH WHITE RICE

Preparation Time: 15 minutes   **Cooking Time**: 3 H   Servings:3

Ingredients:
- 450 grams lamb shoulder
- 2 cups cooked white rice
- 1 ½ cup coconut milk
- 3 garlic cloves, minced
- 1 yellow onion, chopped
- 1 ½ tablespoons chopped ginger
- 2 tablespoons apple cider vinegar
- 1 teaspoon curry powder
- ¼ teaspoon turmeric powder

- ½ teaspoon mustard seeds
- ½ teaspoon ground coriander
- 1 teaspoon ground cumin
- ¼ teaspoon cinnamon powder
- ¼ teaspoon cayenne pepper
- 1 teaspoon salt
- ½ teaspoon ground black pepper
- ½ cup chopped fresh cilantro

Directions:
- Prepare the lamb by cutting it at the bone. Set this aside.
- Pour the coconut milk into the slow cooker. Add in the garlic, onion, ginger and vinegar and mix well.
- Mix the curry powder, turmeric, mustard seeds, coriander, cumin, cinnamon, cayenne, salt and pepper into the coconut milk mixture.
- Place the lamb pieces into the coconut milk and spices and mix well.

- Cover the slow cooker and set the temperature on high. Cook the lamb curry for 3 hours, until the meat separates from the bone.
- Once the meat is cooked, remove the bone pieces and discard.
- Place the cooked white rice on a serving dish
- Spoon the lamb curry and place it on top of the rice, and sprinkle fresh cilantro on top before serving

64. CREAMY BEEF STROGANOFF

Preparation Time: 15 minutes   **Cooking Time**: 4 H   Servings:6

Ingredients:
- 900 grams lean ground beef
- 1 tablespoon olive oil
- 2 cups button mushrooms, halved
- 2 yellow onions, chopped
1 tablespoon minced garlic

- 1 cup coconut milk
- 1 cup plain yoghurt
- 1 cup natural beef stock
- 2 tablespoons gluten free soy sauce
- 2 tablespoons non-gluten mustard
- Pinch of salt and pepper

Directions:
- Heat the olive oil in a large skillet over medium heat
- Fry the ground beef until it becomes slightly brown. Sprinkle some salt and pepper to taste
- Once the beef is cooked, place it inside a large slow cooker.
- Add the mushrooms, onions, garlic, mustard and soy sauce to the ground beef and mix well

- Lastly, pour in the coconut milk and beef stock and cover the slow cooker.
- Set the temperature to high and slow cook the beef for 3 ½ hours
- Once the beef is cooked, pour it into a serving bowl and let it stand for 30 minutes
- Spoon the yoghurt into the stroganoff and mix well before serving

65. GLUTEN FREE VEGAN GUMBO

Preparation Time: 20 minutes   **Cooking Time**: 8 H   Servings:6

Ingredients:

- 1 cup sliced okra
- 1 cup button mushrooms, halved
- 1 red onion, chopped
- 2 celery stalks, chopped
- 1 yellow bell pepper, deseeded and chopped
- 1 zucchini, sliced into quarters
- 1 eggplant, diced
- 3 garlic cloves, chopped
- 2 cups chopped tomatoes
- 2 cups canned kidney beans, washed and drained
- 2 cups water
- 3 tablespoons olive oil
- 2 tablespoons gluten free flour
- 2 tablespoons coconut aminos or non-gluten soy sauce
- 1 tablespoon chili powder
- ½ tablespoon cayenne pepper
- ½ tablespoon salt
- ½ tablespoon ground black pepper
- 3 cups cooked white rice

Directions:

- In a large skillet over medium flame, heat a tablespoon of the olive oil
- Start sautéing the okra, mushrooms, onion, celery, bell pepper, zucchini and eggplant until slightly brown
- Place the sautéed vegetables inside the slow cooker.
- On the same skillet, heat the remaining olive oil and add in the flour
- Stir constantly while slowly pouring in the water
- Allow the water to boil then pour it into the slow cooker.
- Add the tomatoes, kidney beans, coconut aminos, chili powder, cayenne powder, salt and pepper into the slow cooker
- Mix all the ingredients and place a lid on the slow cooker.
- Adjust the cooker's temperature to low and cook the gumbo for 8 hours.
- Place the cooked rice on a serving platter. Pour the cooked gumbo on top of the rice and serve immediately

66. SLOW-COOKED HERB CHICKEN

Preparation Time: 15 minutes   **Cooking Time**: 6 H   Servings:4

Ingredients:

- 7 garlic cloves, minced
- 1 yellow onion, chopped
- 1 carrot, peeled and chopped
- ½ teaspoon sea salt
- ½ teaspoon whole pepper
- 1 teaspoon sage
- 2 teaspoons rosemary
- 1 teaspoon thyme
- 1 whole chicken, neck and insides removed
- 3 cups cooked white rice or quinoa

Directions:

- Rinse the chicken with cold water and drain.
- Place the chopped onions and carrots inside the chicken and the chopped garlic in between the skin and the meat.
- In a small bowl, mix together the salt, pepper, sage, rosemary and thyme
- Rub the spices onto the chicken.
- Place the chicken inside the slow cooker and adjust the temperature to high
- Cover the pot and roast the chicken for 6 hours until the meat falls off the bone.
- Serve this dish with cooked rice or quinoa

67. SLOW COOKER SPICY PORK CHOPS

Preparation Time: 20 minutes   **Cooking Time**: 6 H   **Servings**: 2

Ingredients:
- 4 pork chops
- 1 tablespoon gluten free soy sauce
- 1/3 cup water
- 1 tablespoon olive oil
- 1 cup gluten free ketchup
- 1 teaspoon chili powder
- ½ cup chopped yellow onion
- 2 garlic cloves
- Pinch of salt and pepper

Directions:
- Place a skillet over medium heat and heat the olive oil
- Add the onions to the pan and sauté until it turn light brown.
- Next, add in the garlic, ketchup, soy sauce, salt, pepper, chili powder and water
- Allow the sauce to simmer for 8-10 minutes.
- Place the pork chops inside the slow cooker and pour the sauce over it
- Cover the pot and cook the pork chops on low heat for 6 hours.
- Once the chops are cooked, place them on a serving dish and drizzle the sauce on top

68. HONEY LEMON SALMON AND BROCCOLINI

Preparation Time: 15 minutes   **Cooking Time**: 15 minutes   **Servings**: 4

Ingredients:
- 4 salmon fillets, each about 5 ounces
- 12 ounces Broccolini
- 1 teaspoon ground black pepper
- 1 teaspoon salt
- 1 tablespoons olive oil
- 2 teaspoons sesame seeds

FOR THE HONEY LEMON SAUCE:
- 1 teaspoon minced garlic
- 2 teaspoons cornstarch
- 2 tablespoons soy sauce
- 1/4 cup honey
- 1 tablespoon sesame oil
- 1 lemon, juiced
- 1/4 cup water

Directions:
- Switch on the oven, then set it to 425 degrees F, and let it preheat.
- Place salmon in a large sheet pan, brush it with olive oil, add Broccolini, toss it oil until coated
- Then season with salt and black pepper and bake for 10 minutes.
- In the meantime, prepare the sauce and for this
- Place all its ingredients in a shaker and shake until well combined, and no clumps remain in the sauce.
- When salmon and Broccolini has roasted, drizzle the sauce on them, return the sheet pan into the oven, switch on the broiler
- Continue cooking for 3 to 5 minutes until salmon and Broccolini are nicely browned, rotating the sheet pan halfway through.
- Let the salmon and Broccolini cool, then portion evenly between four heatproof glass meal prep container
- Garnish with sesame seeds.
- Tighten the containers with lid and refrigerate for up to four days or freeze for up to one month.
- When ready to eat, thaw the salmon
- Then reheat the container in the microwave until hot and serve with boiled brown rice

69. TUNA CAKES

Preparation Time: 15 minutes   **Cooking Time:** 16 minutes   **Servings:** 12

Ingredients:

- 24 ounces cooked tuna
- 3/4 cup almond flour
- 1 small onion, peeled, diced
- 2 tablespoons chopped parsley
- 1/4 cup scallions, chopped
- 1/4 cup roasted red peppers, chopped
- 1/2 teaspoon ground black pepper
- 1 teaspoon salt
- 1 teaspoon minced garlic
- 1/2 teaspoon lemon zest
- 1/2 teaspoon paprika
- 1 teaspoon lemon juice

- 1 teaspoon Sriracha sauce
- 1 egg
- 1 egg white

FOR ROASTED RED PEPPER SAUCE:

- 1 cup roasted red pepper
- 3 cloves of garlic, peeled
- 2 tablespoon chopped parsley
- 1/4 teaspoon ground black pepper
- 1/2 teaspoon sea salt
- 1/2 teaspoon cumin
- 1/2 teaspoon smoked paprika
- 1 1/2 tablespoon lemon juice 1/4 cup mayo

Directions:

- Prepare the tuna cakes and for this, place all its ingredients in a large bowl, stir until well combined
- Then shape the mixture into ¾ inch thick patties, about ¼ cup of the tuna mixture per patty.
- Take a large skillet, grease it with oil and when hot, add tuna cakes in a single layer
- Cook for 4 minutes until side until nicely browned on both sides.
- Transfer the tuna cakes to a plate

- Cook the remaining tuna cakes in the same manner, let cool completely.
- Prepare the sauce, and for this, place all its ingredients in a blender and pulse until smooth.
- Portion the cakes evenly between four heatproof glass meal prep containers
- Then portion the sauce separately in the containers.
- Tighten the containers with lid
- Store in the refrigerator for up to four days or freeze for up to two months

70. TUNA SALAD LETTUCE WRAPS

Preparation Time: 15 minutes   **Cooking Time:** 0 minutes   **Servings:** 4

Ingredients:

FOR THE SALAD:

- 8 ounces cooked tuna
- 1 shallot bulb, peeled, diced
- 1/2 dill pickle, diced
- 1 rib of celery, peeled, diced
- 1/4 teaspoon garlic powder
- 1/4 teaspoon sea salt
- 1/4 teaspoon ground black pepper
- 1 tablespoon Dijon mustard

- 2 tablespoons lemon juice
- 2 tablespoons mayonnaise
- 2 tablespoons Greek yogurt

FOR SERVING:

- 6 large romaine lettuce leaves, rinsed
- 2 cups grapes
- 2 medium carrots, peeled, cut into thin strips
- 2 medium cucumbers, cut into thin strips

Directions:

- Place tuna in a bowl, shred it with two forks, then add remaining ingredients and stir until well combined.
- Portion carrots, cucumber, and grapes into four heatproof glass meal prep containers

- Then portion 2 large lettuce leaves into each container and top with 2/3 cup of tuna salad.
- Tighten the containers with lid and refrigerate for up to four days.
- Serve straight away

71. BEEF & BROCCOLI STIR FRY

Preparation Time: 10 minutes   **Cooking Time**: 40 minutes   **Servings:**6

Ingredients:

THE MARINADE:
- Water (.25 cup)
- GF soy sauce (.25 cup)
- Garlic (2 minced)
- Ground pepper (.25 tsp.)
- Boneless round steak/stir-fry beef (1 lb.)

THE STIR FRY:
- Oil (2 tbsp.)
- Broccoli florets (4 cups)
- Onion (.5 cup)
- Carrots (.5 cup)

THEE STIR FRY SAUCE:
- Cold water (1 cup)
- Gluten-free soy sauce (.25 cup)
- Brown sugar (.25 cup)
- Ground ginger (1.5 tsp.)
- Sesame oil (1 tsp.)
- Optional: Red pepper flakes (.25 tsp.)
- Cornstarch (.25 cup)
- Optional: Toasted sesame seeds (1-2 tsp.)
- Optional: Sliced onion greens

Directions:
- Do the prep. Mince the garlic. Thinly slice/chop the onion and carrots. Slice the steak into 3-inch strips.
- Make the marinade
- Whisk the water, soy sauce, garlic, and black Pepper
- Add the stir-fry beef strips and marinate for at least half an hour.
- Stir Fry: In a large frying pan or wok, heat two tablespoons of oil over med-high heat
- Fold in the beef and marinade, and fry until the meat is no longer pink (3-5 min.).
- Then the onions and carrots, and fry, while continuing to stir for another two minutes.
- Join also the broccoli and continue stirring and frying for one more minute.
- In a glass measuring cup, whisk the cup cold water, soy sauce, brown sugar, ginger, sesame oil, red pepper flakes, and cornstarch
- Pour this mixture over the beef & broccoli mixture, and cook until sauce thickens (2-3 min.).
- Serve immediately over hot rice. Sprinkle with toasted sesame seeds and onion greens before serving

72. TACO SEASONING - FOR ONE POUND OF BEEF

Preparation Time: 5 minutes   **Cooking Time**: 5 minutes   **Servings:**1

Ingredients:
- Chili powder (2.5 tsp.)
- Cumin (.75 tsp.)
- Dried oregano (1/8 tsp.)
- Regular/smoked paprika (.25 tsp.)
- Garlic & Onion powder (1/8 tsp. of each)
- Red chili pepper flakes (1/8 tsp.)
- Black pepper and salt (.25 tsp. each)

Directions:
- Whisk each of the seasonings in a mixing container.
- Store in a closed container until it's time to use it

73. CHEESEBURGER CASSEROLE

Preparation Time: 35 minutes   **Cooking Time**: 35 minutes   **Servings:**8

Ingredients:
- Ground beef (2 lb.)
- Large onion (1)
- Shredded cheddar cheese (1 cup)
- Mayo (.25 cup)
- Ketchup (.5 cup)
- Mustard (2 tbsp.)
- GF tater tots - frozen (2 lb.)
- Also Needed: 9x13 baking dish

Directions:
- Set the oven to reach 375° Fahrenheit.
- Chop the onion and shred the cheese.
- Prepare a skillet to cook the onion and beef
- Combine all of the fixings (omit the tater tots).
- Dump the mixture into the dish and add a layer of tater tots.
- Bake it for about half an hour

74. CRUNCHY TACO HAMBURGER HELPER

Preparation Time: 5 minutes   **Cooking Time**: 25 minutes   **Servings**: 5

Ingredients:
- Lean ground beef (1 lb.)
- Large shallot (1) or Small chopped onion (half of one)
- Taco seasoning packet (1 - don't add water)
- Salsa (.5 cup)
- Chicken broth (1.75 cups)
- Long-grain white rice - ex. jasmine/basmati (1 cup)
- Shredded sharp cheddar cheese (1 cup)

SUGGESTED TOPPINGS:
- Additional salsa
- Crushed tortilla chips
- Chopped green onions
- Side of sliced avocado

Directions:
- Prepare a skillet using the med-high temperature setting. Brown the onion and beef
- Mix in the salsa, seasoning, and chicken broth.
- Wait for it to boil
- Stir in the rice and place a lid on the pot. Reduce the heat setting to low.
- Cook slowly until the rice is tender (15-20 min.)
- Remove it from the burner and fold in the cheese until it's melted.
- Place the top back on the pot and wait for five minutes before serving

75. MINI PHILLY CHEESESTEAK MEATLOAVES

Preparation Time: 5 minutes   **Cooking Time**: 30 minutes   **Servings**: 4

Ingredients:
- Butter (1.5 tbsp.)
- Olive oil (1.5 tbsp.)
- Yellow onion (1 small)
- Green pepper (1 small)
- Garlic (2 cloves)
- Black pepper and salt
- Egg (1 whisked)
- Gluten-free Worcestershire sauce (1 tbsp.)
- Lean ground beef (1 lb.)
- Crushed Rice Chex (.5 cup)
- Provolone cheese (3 oz./Cut into ¼-inch cubes)

Directions:
- Set the oven to warm at 425° Fahrenheit
- Cover a baking tray using a layer of foil and a spritz of cooking oil spray.
- Warm the butter and oil in a skillet using the med-high temperature setting
- Mince and sauté the onions and salt until golden (3-4 min.). Dice and add the peppers to sauté (3-4 min.)
- Lower the heat and mince and add the garlic to sauté for about 30 more seconds
- Dump the veggies in a platter to slightly cool.
- Mix the egg, beef, Rice Chex, salt, pepper, Worcestershire sauce, peppers, and onions.
- Divide into four portions to form loaves and place them in the prepared pan. Bake it for about 20-22 min. Serve with your favorite sides

76. DELICIOUS EGG DROP SOUP

Preparation Time: 10minutes   **Cooking Time**: 7 H 15 minutes   **Servings**: 8

Ingredients:
- Chicken broth (1.5 quarts)
- Tapioca flour (2 tbsp. + .25 cup cold water)
- Eggs (2)
- Scallions (2)

Directions:
- Add the broth to a pot to heat
- Once boiling, slowly mix in the tapioca mixture to thicken the broth.
- Slightly whisk the eggs with a fork and lower the heat setting as you mix in the eggs.
- Turn off the heat.
- Chop the scallions and add them to the top to serve

77. FALL LAMB & VEGGIE STEW

Preparation Time: 5 minutes   **Cooking Time:** 7 minutes   Servings:6

Ingredients:
- Lamb stew meat (2 lb.)
- Zucchini (1)
- Summer squash (1)
- Chopped tomatoes (2)
- Mushrooms (1 cup)
- Onions (1 cup)
- Bell peppers (.5 cup)
- A crushed clove of garlic (1)
- Salt (2 tsp.)
- Bay leaf (1)
- Thyme leaves (.5 tsp.)
- Chicken broth (2 cups)

Directions:
- Chop/dice the veggies.
- Toss the lamb and veggies into a crockpot.
- Combine the rest of the fixings and simmer for seven hours using the low-temperature setting

78. GAZPACHO CHILLED SOUP

Preparation Time: 5 minutes   **Cooking Time:** minutes   Servings:4

Ingredients:
- Flaxseed meal (.5 cup)
- Tomatoes (4 cups)
- Bell peppers (1 green & 1 red)
- Cucumber (1)
- Garlic (2 cloves)
- Virgin olive/avocado oil (150 ml)
- Lemon juice (2 tbsp.)

Directions:
- Peel the cucumber and dice it with the peppers and tomatoes
- Mince the garlic. Mix in the oil and flax meal. Blend it until smooth.
- Adjust the salt and lemon juice as preferred.
- Pop it in the fridge to chill.
- Serve the soup with a sprinkle of parsley, mint, black olives, or hard- boiled eggs to your liking.

79. ITALIAN BEEF SOUP

Preparation Time: 5 minutes   **Cooking Time:** 30minutes   Servings:5

Ingredients:
- Minced beef (1 lb.)
- Garlic clove (1)
- Beef broth (2 cups)
- Large tomatoes (2-3 or more if desired)
- Carrots (1 cup)
- Spinach (2 cups)
- Salt & black pepper (.25 tsp. each)

Directions:
- Prep the veggies. Mince the garlic and beef, rinse and tear the spinach, and cube the zucchini
- Slice the carrots.
- Toss and brown the beef in a stockpot using the medium-high temperature setting
- Pour in the broth, tomatoes, carrots, pepper, and salt.
- Lower the heat, place a lid on the pot, and simmer for about 15 minutes.
- Stir in the zucchini and cover to cook the soup until it's tender.
- Add the spinach to wilt for about five minutes before serving

80. JAMBALAYA SOUP

Preparation Time: 10 minutes   **Cooking Time**: 50 minutes   Servings:8

Ingredients:

- Bacon (4 slices)
- GF Andouille sausage/kielbasa (12 oz.)
- Garlic (2 cloves)
- Chicken breasts (2)
- Yellow onion (1 small)
- Celery (2 ribs)
- Bell pepper (1 green)
- Black pepper & salt
- Cajun seasoning (2 tsp.)
- GF flour (3 tbsp.)
- Crushed tomatoes (28 oz.)
- Water (2 cups)
- Bay leaves (2)
- GF Chicken broth (32 oz.)
- Long-grain white rice (.75 cup)
- Also Needed: Six-quart Dutch oven/Heavy-duty soup pot

Directions:

- Chop the bacon, chicken, sausage, bell pepper, onion, and celery. Mince the garlic.
- Add the bacon into the soup pot, setting the temperature on medium - cooking until it's crispy.
- Put the bacon on a platter, reserving the fat, and pour in enough oil to total two tablespoons of fat in the pot.
- Set the temperature at med-high, and add the chicken, salt, and pepper, cooking for about two minutes until it is opaque.
- Chop and add the peppers, celery, onion, and the cajun seasoning.
- Sauté it for about five minutes until they are tender
- Toss in the garlic and continue to sauté them for an additional 30 seconds - or so.
- Dust flour into the pot and simmer the soup for two minutes. Pour in the chicken broth (1-2 splashes at a time)
- Cook for about 15-18 minutes until it's al dente.
- The last two to three minutes, remove the pot from the burner with the lid on to allow the rice time to finish cooking.
- At that time, remove the top and add the bacon. Wait about ten minutes for it to thicken and serve

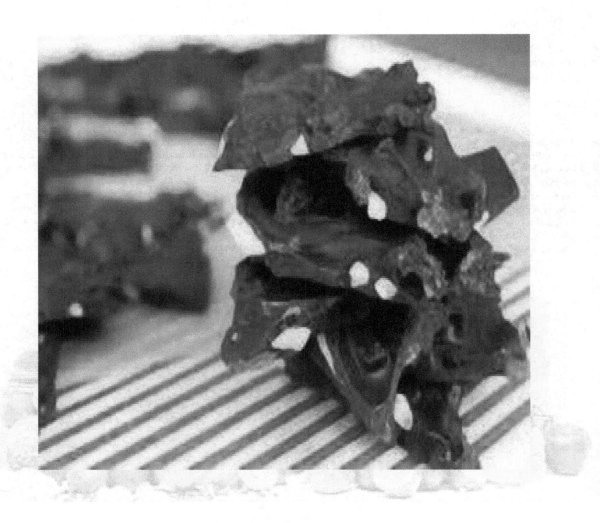

81. OLLAGEN BROWNIE CUPS

Preparation Time: 1 H 10 minutes   **Cooking Time**: 1 minutes   **Servings**:12

Ingredients:
- 1/4 cup almond flour
- 1/2 cup collagen peptides
- 1/4 cup cocoa powder, unsweetened 1 cup chocolate chips
- 1/4 cup peanut butter
- 3 tablespoons maple syrup
- 1/2 cup almond milk, unsweetened

Directions:
- Place 2/3 cup chocolate chips in a heatproof bowl and microwave for 30 seconds until chocolate has melted.
- Take a 12 cups mini muffin pan, line its cups with muffin liner
- Then fill each cup with 1 tablespoon of melted chocolate, swirling it with the back of a spoon and then freeze for 30 minutes until set.
- Meanwhile, prepare the filling and for this
- Place the remaining ingredients in a bowl and mix well until sticky dough comes together.
- Shape the dough into balls and then flatten each ball into discs.
- When the chocolate has set, place dough disc into each muffin cup
- Then flatten it by using fingers to press the disc against the sides of muffin cup.
- Place remaining chocolate chips in a heatproof bowl, microwave for 30 seconds until chocolate has melted
- Then evenly pour the chocolate on dough crust until covered and freeze for another 30 minutes until set.
- Then transfer the cups in a large plastic bag and store in the freezer for up to three months

82. CHOCOLATE ALMOND BARK

Preparation Time: 1 H 10 minutes   **Cooking Time**: 2 minutes   **Servings**:4

Ingredients:
- 1 3/4 cup cacao
- 1/4 cup slivered almonds, unsalted
- 1 tablespoon erythritol sweetener
- 1/4 cup almond butter, unsweetened

Directions:
- Place cacao in a heatproof bowl
- Add butter and sweetener and microwave for 1 to 2 minutes
- (Until cacao and butter have melted, stirring every 30 seconds)
- Take a baking sheet, line it with parchment sheet, then pour the cacao mixture on it
- Spread it evenly with the back of a spoon.
- Sprinkle almond on top of cacao mixture and then freeze for 1 hour until hard.
- Then break it into pieces
- Place the pieces in a large plastic bag, and store in the freezer for up to three months

83. LIME AND AVOCADO TART

Preparation Time: 2H 40 minutes   **Cooking Time** :0 minutes   **Servings**:8

Ingredients:

FOR THE CRUST:
- 1/4 cup shredded coconut, unsweetened
- 1/2 cup chopped pecans
- 1/2 cup chopped dates
- 2 teaspoons lime zest 1/8 teaspoon sea salt

Directions:
- Prepare the crust, and for this
- Place all its ingredients in a food processor and pulse until a sticky paste comes together.
- Spoon the mixture evenly between two mini springform pans
- Spread and press it evenly and then freeze for 30 minutes.
- Meanwhile, prepare the filling, and for this
- Place all its ingredients in a blender and pulse until creamy.

FOR THE TART FILLING:
- 1 1/2 cups avocado puree
- 1/4 cup lime juice
- 1/4 cup honey
- 1 tablespoon coconut oil
- 1 teaspoon lime zest

- Take out the frozen crusts from the freezer, pour half of the filling in one pan and the other half of filling in the second pan
- Smooth the top, and continue freezing for a minimum of 2 hours.
- Then wrap each tart in plastic wrap and freeze for up to three months.
- When ready to eat, let the tart sit at room temperature for 15 minutes, then cut it into slices and serve

84. BROWNIES

Preparation Time: 15 minutes   **Cooking Time**: 0 minutes   **Servings**:8

Ingredients:
1 cup vanilla almonds, honey roasted
2 tablespoons cocoa powder

20 Medjool dates, pitted
1 tablespoon water

Directions:
- Place the almonds in a food processor, pulse until coarsely chopped
- Tip the almonds into a bowl and then set aside until required.
- Add dates in the food processor, pulse until coarsely chopped
- Then cocoa powder and water, and pulse again until the dough comes together.

- Join also almonds, pulse again until incorporated
- Transfer the dough in a large bowl and knead for 3 minutes until smooth.
- Place a large piece of parchment paper on a clean working space, place dough on it, and roll it into 1/3-inch thick slab.
- Use a knife to cut squares from the dough, about eight
- Wrap each brownie in plastic wrap and store in the freezer for up to three months

85. BLUEBERRY CUSTARD PIE

Preparation Time: 1H 20 minutes   **Cooking Time**: 8 minutes   Servings:6

Ingredients:

FOR THE CRUST:
- 1 cup walnuts
- 2 cups dates, pitted
- 1/4 cup shredded coconut, unsweetened
- 1 cup almonds

FOR THE FILLING:
- 3 tablespoons cornstarch
- 2/3 cup coconut sugar

- 1 teaspoon vanilla extract, unsweetened
- 1 tablespoon coconut oil
- 2 cups vanilla Almond Breeze, unsweetened

FOR THE TOPPING:
- 2 tablespoons blueberry jam 1
- 1/2 cups fresh blueberries

Directions:

- Prepare the crust, and for this, place all its ingredients in a food processor and pulse until ground.
- Take a 9 inches round pan with a removable bottom, grease it with oil, spoon in crust mixture
- Spread and press it evenly into the pan, set aside until required.
- Prepare the filling and for this, take a pot, add cornstarch and coconut sugar
- Stir in mixed and then whisk in the almond breeze until combined.
- Place the pot over medium-high heat, bring the mixture to boil, then reduce heat to low level
- Cook for 5 minutes until the mixture has thickened, whisking continuously.
- Remove the pot from heat, whisk in vanilla and oil until combined, then pour the filling into the crust, smooth the top and let cool.
- Then wrap the pan tightly with a plastic wrap
- Refrigerate for 1 hour, and then store in the freezer for up to three months.
- When ready to eat, let the pie rest for 20 minutes at room temperature, then cut out a slice
- Top it with blueberry jam and blueberries and serve

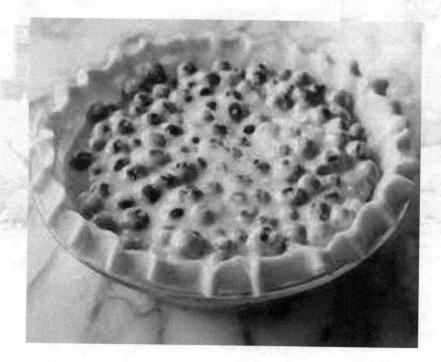

86. MATCHA COCONUT TARTS

Preparation Time: 20 minutes   **Cooking Time:** 26 minutes   **Servings:2**

Ingredients:

FOR THE CRUST:
- ¼ cup shredded coconut, unsweetened
- ½ cup oat flour
- ½ cup buckwheat flour
- 4 teaspoons tapioca starch
- 1/8 teaspoon salt
- 3 tablespoons maple syrup
- 2 tablespoons cacao powder

3 tablespoons melted coconut oil

FOR THE FILLING:
- ½ cup cashews, soaked
- ½ teaspoon agar powder
- 2 teaspoons matcha powder
- ¼ cup maple syrup
- 1 cup coconut cream
- ¼ cup water

Directions:
- Switch on the oven, then set it to 345 degrees F, and let it preheat.
- Meanwhile, prepare the crust, and for this, place oats in a food processor along with coconut and pulse until ground.
- Tip the mixture in a large bowl, add buckwheat flour, cacao, salt, and tapioca starch
- Stir well until mixed, then gradually mix oil and maple syrup using your fingers until dough comes together, set aside for 10 minutes.
- Then take two ramekins, grease them with oil, and line the bottom with baking paper.
- Divide the prepared dough into two portions, place each portion in a ramekin
- Spread and press it in the base and sides of ramekin and bake for 16 minutes on the middle shelf of oven, let them cool completely.

- Meanwhile, prepare the filling and for this
- Place cashews in a food processor, add maple syrup, matcha, and coconut cream and blend until smooth.
- Take a small pot, place it over medium heat, pour in water, stir in agar powder, bring the mixture to boil
- Then switch heat to medium-low level and simmer for 15 minutes until agar has dissolved
- Let the mixture cool for 10 minutes.
- Pour the agar mixture into the food processor and pulse for 1 minute until smooth.
- Evenly divide the filling between two ramekins, smooth the top and refrigerate for 30 minutes until tarts have set.
- Wrap each tart in plastic wrap and store in the refrigerator for up to five days or freeze for up to one month

87. SLOW-COOKED BANANAS FOSTER

Preparation Time: 15 minutes   **Cooking Time:** 2 H   **Servings:5**

Ingredients:
- 5 bananas, peeled and sliced
- 1 cup coconut sugar
- 4 tablespoons melted butter

- ½ cup chopped almonds
- ¼ cup rum
- ½ teaspoon cinnamon powder
- ½ cup grated coconut

Directions:
- In a small bowl, mix together the coconut sugar, butter, rum and cinnamon. Set this aside.
- Arrange the banana slices inside the slow cooker. Pour the sugar and rum mixture on top of the bananas and cover it.

- Cook the bananas on low heat for 2 hours. Sprinkle the coconut and almonds on top within the last 15 minutes of cooking.
- Serve this dessert by itself or with a scoop of vanilla ice cream

88. SCRUMPTIOUS CRÈME BRULEE

Preparation Time: 10 minutes   **Cooking Time**: 4 H   **Servings:**4

Ingredients:
- 5 egg yolks
- ½ cup white sugar
- ¼ cup raw sugar
- 2 cups whipping cream
- 1 tablespoon vanilla

Directions:
- In a large bowl, whip the egg yolks while slowly adding the white sugar and whipping cream
- Add in the vanilla and mix well.
- Place the crème brulee mixture in a baking dish that will fit inside the slow cooker. Set this aside.
- To create a water bath for the crème brulee, pour some water into the slow cooker
- Place the baking dish with the crème brulee mixture inside of it
- Make sure that the water is halfway up the top of the baking dish.
- Cover the slow cooker. Set the temperature to high and cook the crème brulee for 4 hours.
- After 4 hours, turn off the slow cooker and remove the baking dish. Let the dessert cool for 30 minutes
- Sprinkle the raw sugar on top
- Then slightly brown it with a handy butane torch to create a crisp topping. Serve immediately.

89. SLOW COOKER CARAMELIZED PEACHES

Preparation Time: 20 minutes   **Cooking Time**: 2 H   **Servings:**10

Ingredients:
- 10 peaches, peeled, pitted and sliced
- ½ cup butter
- 1 cup coconut sugar
- ½ teaspoon powdered cloves
- ½ teaspoon cinnamon powder
- Scoop of gluten free ice cream

Directions:
- Place peaches, butter, coconut sugar, cloves and cinnamon in a slow cooker and mix.
- Set the temperature to low
- Cover the slow cooker
- Leave the peaches to caramelize for 2 hours then turn off the heat.
- To arrange this dessert, divide the peaches into individual bowls and place a scoop of ice cream on top. Serve immediately

90. BANANA BREAD PUDDING

Preparation Time: 15 minutes   **Cooking Time**: 2 H   **Servings:**5

Ingredients:
- 5 bananas, peeled and chopped
- 6 cups cubed gluten free bread
- ½ cup maple syrup
- ½ cup granulated sugar
- ½ cup toasted pecans Pinch of salt
- 1 teaspoon brandy or rum
- ½ teaspoon minced ginger
- ½ teaspoon cinnamon powder
- ½ teaspoon nutmeg
- ½ cup almond milk 1 teaspoon butter

Directions:
- In a mixing bowl, combine the sugar, pecans, brandy and bananas.
- Mix them well and set it aside.
- In a separate bowl, mix together the almond milk, maple syrup, ginger, cinnamon, nutmeg and salt
- Pour in the cubed bread and coat it with the milk mixture. Set this aside as well.
- Lightly grease the bottom of the slow cooker with butter
- Slowly pour in a half of the milk and bread mixture into the pot then spoon one half of the banana mixture on top of it
- Repeat the same order of layering. Cover the pot and set the temperature to high.
- Cook the bread pudding for an hour and 45 minutes
- Once the pudding is firm, turn off the slow cooker and serve it while it's hot

91. SLICED PEARS WITH GOOEY BUTTERSCOTCH SAUCE

Preparation Time: 10 minutes   **Cooking Time**: 1 H 10 minutes   **Servings**:4

Ingredients:
- 2 apples, cored and sliced
- 2 ¾ cup butterscotch chips
-
- 1 tablespoon rum
- ½ cup evaporated milk
- ½ cup finely chopped almonds

Directions:
- Place the milk and butterscotch chips in a slow cooker, cover it and cook on low heat for 1 hour
- Stir the butterscotch sauce every 15 minutes.
- After an hour, turn off the slow cooker
- Add the rum and chopped almonds into the butterscotch and mix well
- Pour the prepared butterscotch in a sauce bowl.
- Arrange the apple slices on the sides of a serving dish
- Place the butterscotch sauce at the middle or dunk a few pieces of fruit into the sauce. Serve immediately

92. HOMEMADE CHOCOLATE FUDGE

Preparation Time: 5 minutes   **Cooking Time**: 8 H 10 minutes   **Servings**:5

Ingredients:
- ¼ cup coconut milk
- 2 ½ cup dark chocolate chips
- ¼ cup raw honey
- 1 teaspoon vanilla extract Pinch of sea salt

Directions:
- Place the milk, chocolate chips, honey, vanilla and salt in a slow cooker and mix well.
- Cover the pot and set the temperature to low. Cook the fudge for 2 hours but do not stir it.
- After 2 hours, turn off the slow cooker and uncover it. Lightly stir the fudge then leave it to cool for 3 hours.
- Once the fudge has reached room temperature, use a wooden spoon to beat it for 10 minutes
- Pour the fudge into a greased dish, cover it with plastic wrap then place it in a freezer for 3 hours.
- Slice the chocolate fudge into squares before serving

93. SLOW COOKER CARAMEL APPLES

Preparation Time: 15 minutes   **Cooking Time**: 1 H   **Servings**:6

Ingredients:
- 6 red apples, preferably Fuji or Gala variants
- 2 cups caramel candy cubes
- ¼ cup water
- Pinch of salt
- Popsicle sticks and wax paper

Directions:
- Wash the apples and remove the stems
- Pierce a popsicle stick halfway through each of the apples. Set this aside.
- Place the caramel candies, salt and water inside a slow cooker.
- Cover it and cook the caramel on high for one hour.
- Turn off the slow cooker and uncover it
- Dip each apple into the caramel sauce, let the excess drip and place it on a sheet of wax paper to cool

94. CHOCOLATE CHIA PUDDING

Preparation Time: 25 minutes   **Cooking Time**: 0 minutes   **Servings**:1

Ingredients:

- 2 tablespoons chia seeds
- 1 tablespoon cacao powder
- 1/2 teaspoon vanilla extract, unsweetened
- 1 tablespoon maple syrup
- 1/2 cup milk
- Fresh strawberries as needed for topping
- Shredded coconut as needed for topping

Directions:

- Take a small glass jar, place chia seeds in it, ass cocoa powder, pour in milk
- Stir well and let it rest for 15 minutes.
- Stir the chia seeds again
- Then stir in vanilla and maple syrup
- Top with strawberries and coconut.
- Tighten the jar with the lid and store the pudding in the refrigerator for up to three days or freeze for up to one month

95. RICE CRISPY TREATS

Preparation Time:1 H 10 minutes   **Cooking Time**: 0 minutes   **Servings**:12

Ingredients:

- 4 cups brown rice crisp cereal
- 2 tablespoons chocolate chips
- ⅔ cup brown rice syrup
- 1/8 teaspoon salt
- 1/2 teaspoon vanilla extract, unsweetened
- 1 tablespoon coconut oil
- 1/4 cup almond butter

Directions:

- Place the brown rice cereal in a large bowl and set aside until required.
- Take a saucepan, place it over medium heat, add oil, butter, and brown rice syrup, stir well
- Cook for 5 minutes until creamy.
- Remove the pan from heat, whisk in salt and vanilla
- Then pour the mixture over cereal and stir until well combined.
- Take a square baking dish, line it with parchment paper, transfer prepared cereal on it
- Spread and press in the base by using your hands.
- Top the cereal with chocolate chips, press into the cereal, and refrigerate for 1 hour.
- Then cut the cereal into squares, wrap each square in plastic wrap
- Store in refrigerator for up to one week or freeze for up to two months

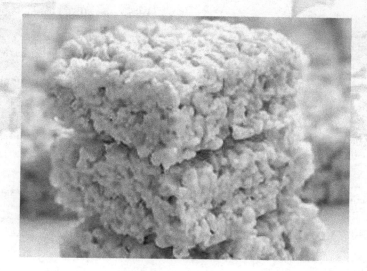

96. BANANA DATE PIE

Preparation Time: 5 H   **Cooking Time:** 20 minutes   **Servings:**4

Ingredients:

CRUST
- 1 & ½ cups blanched almond flour
- 5 large dates, finely chopped
- Fine sea salt, a large pinch
- 3 tbsp coconut or grape seed oil

FILLING
- 5 small ripe bananas cut into pieces
- 5 large medjool dates, chopped
- 1 cup coconut milk, light and unsweetened
- 1/ 3 cup unsweetened cocoa powder, measured then sifted
- 1 tbsp. pure vanilla extract
- ½ cup sliced almonds
- 2 oz. dark chocolate, chopped or shaved

Directions:
- Coat a 9-in. pie plate with nonstick spray.
- Preheat oven to 350ºF (180ºC). In a food processor, add dates, salt and almond flour. Pulsate until thoroughly combined.
- Add oil; mix until dough begins to form. If needed, put an additional few drops.
- Bake until the crust color turns brown, a minimum of 12 - 15 minutes

- Put to one side so it cools and hardens.
- Filling :In a food processor combine coconut milk, dates, cocoa powder, vanilla and
- bananas and pulsate
- When you have a smooth thickness, dispense mix on pie crust.
- Garnish with chocolate that's shaved off with a potato peeler and sliced almonds.
- Wrap with plastic wrap; put in refrigerator a minimum of 4 hrs. Before serving, remove from refrigerator for a minimum of ½ hr

97. GAZPACHO CHILLED SOUP

Preparation Time: 5 minutes   **Cooking Time:** 20 minutes   **Servings:**4

Ingredients:
- Flaxseed meal (.5 cup)
- Tomatoes (4 cups)
- Bell peppers (1 green & 1 red)

- Cucumber (1)
- Garlic (2 cloves)
- Virgin olive/avocado oil (150 ml)
- Lemon juice (2 tbsp.)

Directions:
- Peel the cucumber and dice it with the peppers and tomatoes
- Mince the garlic. Mix in the oil and flax meal. Blend it until smooth.

- Adjust the salt and lemon juice as preferred.
- Pop it in the fridge to chill.
- Serve the soup with a sprinkle of parsley, mint, black olives, or hard- boiled eggs to your liking

98. BLUEBERRY POMEGRANATE SMOOTHIE

Preparation Time: 15 minutes   **Cooking Time:** 0 minutes   **Servings:**1

Ingredients:
- 2/3 cup frozen blueberries (unthawed)
- ½ cup fat-free French vanilla yogurt (we used Stonyfield)

- 1/3 cup vanilla coconut milk
- ¼ cup pomegranate juice

Directions:
- Into a blender, add ¼ cup pomegranate juice, 1/3 cup soy milk

- Then ½ cup yogurt and 2/3 cup unthawed frozen blueberries.
- Turn blender on the highest setting until smooth

99. GINGER BLUEBERRY PARFAIT

Preparation Time: 15 minutes   **Cooking Time**: 0 minutes   Servings:4

Ingredients:
- 1 c blueberries
- 1 tsp grated peeled fresh ginger
- 4 Tbsp maple syrup, divided
- 1 Hass avocado, peeled, pitted, and chopped
- 1 c part-skim ricotta cheese
- 4 sprigs fresh mint

Directions:
- In a small bowl thoroughly mix 1 Tbsp maple syrup, ginger and blueberries. Set to one side 5 minutes.
- In the meantime, put avocado, ricotta, and the rest of the maple syrup, ricotta and avocado in a food processor. Puree ingredients.
- Spoon ricotta mixture, then blueberry mixture interchangeably into 4 dessert dishes or parfait glasses; end with berries.
- Add mint sprigs for beauty.

100. KIWI BLUEBERRY TART

Preparation Time: 10 minutes   **Cooking Time**: 25 minutes   Servings:4

Ingredients:
- 2 store-bought GF pie doughs
- 4 mini tart pans
- 2/3 cup reduced-fat sour cream
- 1 tbsp light brown sugar
- 1¼ cups quartered sliced kiwifruit
- ¼ cup blueberries

Directions:
- Preheat oven to 375°F (190°C).
- Open pie doughs; cut into four 5½"-diameter circles.
- Push into four 4 3/4"-diameter mini tart pans with removable bottoms.
- With a fork, prick the dough, then freeze for 10 minutes, till firm.
- Remove from freezer. Using foil, line tart shells with dried beans or pie weights.
- Bake about 10 minutes until golden. Take dried beans or pie weights off.
- Bake about 4 minutes until golden brown. Allow to sit at room temperature until thoroughly cooled.
- Mix 1 Tbsp light brown sugar and 2/3 cup reduced-fat sour cream.
- Take the shells out of the pie pans. Spoon sour cream mix on top, then add blueberries and kiwi fruit

Thanks for reading this book

CPSIA information can be obtained
at www.ICGtesting.com
Printed in the USA
BVHW062013190521
607713BV00007B/524

9 781802 942179